"I wish I had had such guidance when I was delivering babies. If you are pregnant or contemplating pregnancy, you need this book . . . a lot of good practical advice for all mothers."

JOHN R. LEE, M.D., AUTHOR, *What Your Doctor May Not Tell You About Menopause*

Dean Raffelock, D.C., Dipl. Ac., C.C.N.

Robert Rountree, M.D.

and Virginia Hopkins *with*

Melissa Block

Avery

a member of

Penguin Putnam Inc.

New York

A Natural
Guide to
Pregnancy and
Postpartum
Health

Most Avery books are available at special quantity discounts for bulk purchase for sales promotions, premiums, fund-raising, and educational needs. Special books or book excerpts also can be created to fit specific needs. For details, write Putnam Special Markets, 375 Hudson Street, New York, NY 10014.

a member of
Penguin Putnam Inc.
375 Hudson Street
New York, NY 10014
www.penguinputnam.com

Copyright © 2002 by Dr. Dean Raffelock
All rights reserved. This book, or parts thereof, may not
be reproduced in any form without written permission.
Published simultaneously in Canada

Library of Congress Cataloging-in-Publication Data

Raffelock, Dean.
A natural guide to pregnancy and postpartum health / Dean Raffelock,
Robert Rountree, and Virginia Hopkins ; with Melissa Block.
p.   cm.
Includes bibliographical references and index.
ISBN 1-58333-138-7
1. Pregnancy—Nutritional aspects.   2. Mothers—Nutrition.   3. Postnatal care.
4. Holistic medicine.   I. Rountree, Robert.   II. Title.
RG559.R34   2002   2002071212
618.2'4—dc21

Printed in the United States of America
1 3 5 7 9 10 8 6 4 2

Book design by Meighan Cavanaugh

Acknowledgments

My first acknowledgment goes to my loving wife, Stephanie, for passionately bringing to me the idea for this book, helping me to see some of these key health issues from a woman's perspective, and convincing me that this was a book that needed to be written. You are truly a great wife, partner, playmate, lover, spiritual companion, and best friend. I love you dearly.

So many thanks to Virginia Hopkins for her largeness of spirit for taking on this book project when she really needed a well-deserved vacation. Deep thanks to Melissa Block for extraordinary research, attention to detail, inspired writing, and input from her "new mother's perspective."

Both Virginia Hopkins and I would like to thank Sri Gary and Joy Olsen for teaching us that the soul in us all is eternal, loved, and a true spark of the Divine. For the deep inspiration and spiritual guidance, mere words cannot express our deepest gratitude for the many blessings so generously gifted.

Thanks to Bob Rountree, M.D., for being the kind of physician who is thoroughly grounded in Western medicine and is truly open to the healing power of herbs, nutrition, and good psychology. You are an inspiration and hopefully a prototype of the medical doctor of the future.

To David Luce, M.D., for being such a warmhearted, steadfast medical ally and supporter all these years. You are my spiritual brother.

To Jay Wilson, D.C., for inspiring me to learn about herbs and to become a better nutritionist, and for always being there for me when I needed a chiropractic treatment.

To George Goodheart, D.C., the founder and developer of applied kinesiology, for helping me to understand how the different systems of the human body interact. To Walter Schmidt, D.C., for helping me to understand many of the links between the nervous system, endocrine system, and nutritional biochemistry. To David S. Walther, D.C., for helping me to understand the importance of being a really thorough structural doctor and for tireless work in organizing applied kinesiology. To Jeff Band, Ph.D., for tireless years of championing functional medicine and teaching me the value of research-based nutritional biochemistry. To Bob Lerman, M.D., and David Jones, M.D., for embracing and carrying out a vision of functional medicine that respects all medical disciplines. To Emmett Smith, Dipl.Ac., for teaching me acupuncture in a way that truly made sense and for encouraging me to study for and pass my acupuncture diplomate boards. To Winna Henry for forming the International and American Association of Clinical Nutritionists (IAACN) and for "keeping the flame burning."

To the memory of my father, Abe, who couldn't realize his dream to become a doctor but so generously helped me to realize mine. Thanks for believing in your son. To my mother, Ethel, brother Robert, and brother Dennis; thanks for all the lessons taught and learned.

To Dena Kaye for your enduring and always generous friendship.

Thanks so very much to all the people who became patients and trusted me to participate in their health care these past twenty-five years. Thanks for teaching me how to listen and for inspiring me to keep learning. Your faith in me taught me to have faith in myself.

And to you, the reader: Thanks so much for your interest in the information provided in this book. My fondest hope is that it may enhance your health and enjoyment of life in some way. This book represents a collaboration between a conventionally trained medical doctor and a chiropractor/acupuncturist/nutritionist. Both of us have sought much knowledge beyond the usual scope of traditional M.D. and D.C. practices in order to be able to more comprehensively care for the whole person. May the walls between the different medical professions quickly dissolve so that people everywhere can receive health care that represents the best merging of conventional and holistic medicine.

—D.R.

Contents

Preface

In the 1950s, countless women thought they were being helped through menopause by modern medicine. These women underwent hysterectomies that were performed as a therapeutic aid for "calming them down." The word *hysterectomy* has its root in the Latin word *hysteria,* so we might as well have called them "hysteria-ectomies." Today, we know that women experience profound hormonal changes during menopause and alternative medicine is more likely to ease their discomfort with carefully and individually prescribed natural hormone replacement rather than with radical surgery.

Yet in this new century, countless women who have just had babies are being medicated with Prozac, Paxil, Zoloft, Celexa, and the like. Modern medicine wants to help calm them down because it appears that some of these women cannot cope. Yet what we are learning today is that many forms of postpartum depression and anxiety have their roots in nutritional and hormonal depletion. Depletion of these vital physiological substances can produce powerful emotional and physiological imbalances and can have long-term negative effects even decades later if not treated properly.

This is a book about the need for "pregnancy recovery"—the need for adequate rest, a healthy diet, and nutritional therapy after childbirth to help rebuild the mother's vital nutrient reserves, which were donated to form her new baby's entire body. Pregnancy recovery also introduces the notion that mothers who replenish their energy reserves after giving birth ultimately make better mothers and are more likely to be able to give birth again, if they so desire, without sacrificing their own health or the health of any future children.

The issue of pregnancy recovery is not far removed from what the menopausal women of the 1950s experienced, except that the issue here is one of physiological support rather than emotional control. Most women need to realize that it is okay, even desirable, to take care of themselves after giving birth. There seems to be a myth in this country that a woman can pop out a baby on Tuesday and be "back in the field" plowing on Wednesday. Let's not forget that it took a mandate of Congress to provide that insurance companies allow women to stay in the hospital for forty-eight hours after a normal vaginal birth, rather than sending them home in twenty-four hours. If a woman does get anxious or depressed after giving birth, the conventional medical "wisdom" is to medicate her with powerful and potentially dangerous drugs, rather than to understand that her body has just donated a tremendous amount of its nutrient reserves to form the body of her baby, and that replenishing these nutrients is the first area in her health care that should be addressed.

Pregnancy recovery—the kind that is supported by employers who give adequate leaves of absence for the postpartum period, doctors who recognize the need for nutritional rebuilding, and families who understand that new mothers need rest in order to become rejuvenated—is a political issue and a health-care issue, as well as an issue of consciousness. All of us ache when we pick up the paper and read about a mother who harmed or even killed her child because she was depressed. This is most likely a mother who had too many babies in too short a time period, without the rest and nutritional support needed to help her body recover after pregnancy. Pregnancy recovery is an idea whose time has come. It is our hope that this book will help to raise awareness of this issue and lead to its receiving the kind of attention it deserves.

This book is dedicated to moms everywhere!

How to Use This Book

In our hustling, bustling, youth-oriented, sex-obsessed culture, the processes of pregnancy, birth, and pregnancy recovery receive a great deal less attention than the processes that get women pregnant in the first place. It is no wonder that so many women suffer from emotional and physical ailments after giving birth: they are undergoing an enormous life change at a time when their bodies are probably more depleted than they have ever been, and our culture barely acknowledges their struggles except to say they are "par for the course."

Every woman needs to take care of herself following a pregnancy. There are no superwomen who don't need some extra support during this trying time. If you are dealing with postpartum depression or any other postpartum problem, you may feel as though there is no space in your life to do the work of healing yourself. If you are caring for a baby, you certainly don't have the energy to embark on a complicated self-improvement program—or even to read this entire book!

With this in mind, we have designed this book so that you can benefit from each chapter individually if you don't have the time to read it from cover to cover. You can even use the index to target specific problems and solutions if you don't have the time to read an entire chapter at one time.

If you are reading this book while you are pregnant, congratulations on your foresight and commitment to supporting your own health and the health of your baby. Learn as much as you can before your baby's arrival, and you will be prepared to deal with problems as soon as they begin to arise.

There are many lifestyle choices a woman can make to support both herself and her baby. Even making the most basic sound nutritional choices can mean the difference between depression and fatigue or well-being and bountiful energy. In these pages, we will give you the benefit of our joint medical and nutritional expertise to help you make the choices that work for you.

1

I Have a Beautiful Baby.
Why Do I Feel So Terrible?

A friend of ours says that when she was about six months along in her pregnancy, it seemed as if every woman in her life who had ever been pregnant—from her mother to her friends, cousins, and coworkers—began recounting their worst horror stories about pregnancy. However, when her water broke and she went into labor, it began to dawn on her that no amount of shared experience could ever prepare her for what is one of the most intense, intimate rites of passage in a woman's life: the initiation into motherhood. Birthing a baby runs the gamut from the intensity of the physical to the sublime of the spiritual, whether it is your first baby or your fifth.

Then there is another story that is so common, yet hardly ever talked about. That's the story of what it is like after you have had a baby—the story of the largely unspoken need for pregnancy recovery. Once that baby is born, all eyes are upon your little creation.

You go to the doctor and are asked, "How are you feeling?" You start to answer, "Okay . . . ," and before you can say another word, the attention turns to the baby. "How is your baby eating? How is your baby sleeping? How much weight has she gained?" and so forth. A well-meaning grandmother will tell you, "Why sweetheart, it's all about your baby." And wanting to be a good mom, maybe you begin to think that some of those aches and pains, some of those hard-to-sort-out emotions, some of that exhaustion or anxiety that you have felt since childbirth aren't really so important. It's all about the baby, right? Does being a good mother mean taking care of your baby at the expense of yourself?

Ever since your bundle of joy was conceived, you have been doing all you can for your little one. Perhaps you were one of those women who strictly followed all of the dietary advice given in pregnancy and childbirth books. You probably took the prenatal vitamins prescribed by your doctor and gave up that glass of wine with dinner. You most likely listened to advice from your mother, your coworkers, and even the woman at the supermarket checkout counter. In short, you have done everything you could to ensure your baby's good health and safe passage into the world.

Still, a lot of women experience quite a few surprises during the hard work of giving birth. Some find that their bodies hurt in ways unimagined. Sometimes that carefully detailed birth plan turns out not to be the way it all pans out. There is no way to prepare or know for sure what it is like to push life out of your body into the world. In the aftermath, you are likely to feel much older and certainly much wiser, as you have learned something you could never explain to someone who hasn't been there. You have entered the ranks of motherhood, and life is going to be very different from now on.

To you, your baby is now, and will hereafter be, perfect. And yet, in between your feelings of intense, glowing love, pride, and fulfillment, you may be feeling not just tired or fatigued, but exhausted. You may also be feeling discouraged, fearful, terribly insecure, or even depressed. Your belly may still look as though there might be another baby in there, except for the fact that it jiggles when you move. If you are breastfeeding, your breasts may often become so engorged that they feel like overfull sandbags propped on your chest. There is a good chance that you are constipated or that you are having headaches for the first time in your life. Your back may be killing you, and you may feel like telling your husband, "Don't even think about touching me." What's going on?

You're Postpartum but Not Picture-Perfect

Birth is a celebrated event, much anticipated and prepared for by most mothers. Months of prenatal care lead up to that first labor pang—the one that tells the mother that the time to have her baby has finally arrived. Her journey from that point forward depends on many factors, including her chosen approach to birth (natural or otherwise), where she has her baby (home, birthing center, or hospital), the people she has chosen to support her, and her own ability to endure the discomfort of labor and childbirth.

Birth experiences are incredibly varied. Some women find the whole process easier than they expected, giving birth after only a few short hours of labor and two or three pushes. Others experience many hours of labor before giving birth. Most who give birth in a hospital choose to have epidural anesthesia, which makes the whole experience a lot less painful—but, some argue, makes it more likely that there will be further medical intervention. Some birthing moms need cesarean section (C-section) or other forms of medical assistance. No matter how well childbirth goes, it is still the physical (and sometimes the emotional) equivalent of running two marathons back to back. In the end, the most important thing is that mother and baby are well.

Many first-time mothers find themselves traumatized by their birth experiences, but once they are busy with the task of caring for a newborn, they don't have the opportunity to process what they've just been through. After the work of giving birth is done, the stress on the mother only increases. When we talk about stress, we are describing a state in which your body is on more or less constant overdrive. On little sleep, and with a body that has been through a great challenge, you face the task of caring for your newborn baby. Where do the resources for accomplishing this stressful transition from pregnant woman to new mother come from? They are drawn from the nutrients that make up your tissues and enter your body in the form of food. That's right: You are what you eat, and the food you eat is what enables you to get up every morning and do what needs to be done. Every cell, every organ, every muscle, every bone, every fluid in your body is made up of the stuff you eat and drink. During pregnancy, your body must also supply the raw materials for the cells, organs, tissues, and fluids that make up your new bundle of joy. For mothers who breastfeed, this relationship continues with your child until he weans.

Breastfeeding is a continuous drain on the protein, fat, and mineral reserves of the mother's body. Many women breastfeed their babies for six months to a year, and some do so for up to three years. Sleep deprivation, managing life with an infant, and, perhaps, returning to work within a matter of weeks all collaborate to further deplete nutrient reserves. Stress itself uses up more of all the nutrients needed to keep the body working smoothly, particularly the B vitamins, vitamin C, essential fatty acids, and key minerals like zinc and magnesium.

A woman who has been careful about her diet during pregnancy may fall off the wagon after the baby is born. Nursing mothers often have enormous appetites. Yet a diet high in refined carbohydrates, sugars, and unhealthy fats such as those found in fried foods will actually rob a mother's body of vital nutrients. Unless the mother's nutrient reserves are replenished, she is likely to have postpregnancy symptoms that will baffle most physicians.

New mothers routinely suffer from low immunity, weight problems, back pain, and gastrointestinal troubles. Emotional ups and downs are par for the course, and these—along with the loss of libido that is most pronounced in breastfeeding mothers—can create strife between the mother and her partner. If a woman has had a traumatic birthing experience, she may need months of supportive attention to recover.

Most women complain of foggy thinking and memory loss after giving birth, and many fight off terrifying thoughts of hurting or abandoning their babies. Colicky or especially demanding infants can drive even the most loving mothers to desperation. On top of all of this, a new mother's life tends to be a lonely one. If she is living in a one-family household with only her partner and child, without family or close friends around, the loneliness of new motherhood can be overwhelming.

Throughout this book, you will read about women who have been where you find yourself today. Some of them are our patients, and their stories have been included to give you real-life examples of how our pregnancy recovery program helped them and can help you. Other stories have been included simply to let you know that *you are not alone* in your experiences. Sometimes women in the throes of postpartum difficulties simply need to know that their experiences are valid and real, and that time and perspective will carry them through. The key concepts to understand are that your newborn baby's body is entirely formed from nutrients donated from your body's nutrient reserves, and that, if these nutrient depletions are not replenished, your chances of having postpartum symptoms greatly increase. If these nutrient depletions are not identified and replenished, symptoms may last for years or even decades.

One woman told us that she had had constant thoughts of hurting her newborn baby. Every time she saw a sharp knife on the counter, walked along a steep drop, or stood next to a body of water, she could not stop thinking about hurting her baby. Her thoughts frightened her and she wondered if she was an unfit parent. Finally, she confided her thoughts to another mother. "You're kidding!" exclaimed the other mom. "I have exactly those same thoughts. I'm so relieved that I'm not the only one!" They talked about it and decided that these thoughts were not signs that they desired to hurt their babies, but that they were so afraid of harm coming to them that their minds raced to the worst possible scenario as soon as any danger appeared. Once they acknowledged those thoughts and feelings, they both felt much better.

Building the Case for a Pregnancy Recovery Program

Many women have observed that they started to suffer from various symptoms shortly after giving birth. Many of them believe that they have postpartum depression, but other symptoms are just as commonly mentioned.

The complaints that tend to appear in women soon after giving birth are many and varied, and include the following:

- Allergies.
- Asthma.
- Back, pelvic, or neck pain.
- Chronic bladder infections.
- Chronic fatigue.
- Depression, anxiety, and/or irritability.
- Digestive disturbances.
- Dizziness/vertigo.
- Hair loss or weak, brittle nails.
- Insomnia.
- Irritable bowel syndrome.
- Joint pain.
- Loss of sex drive.
- Lowered immunity (manifested by "catching every cold or flu that comes around").
- Muscle weakness.
- Pounding headaches.
- Rapid heart rate.
- Skin problems.
- Unexplained sadness (often expressed as "crying for no reason").
- Yeast infections.

Even moms whose youngest children are over twenty-five years old still often remember their symptoms as having begun soon after they gave birth. This raises the question of why so many women begin to have such a wide variety of symptoms shortly after pregnancy.

We believe that the key to finding the common thread that links so many women lies in the mysteries of *biochemical nutrition*—the study of nutritional building blocks as they relate to the form and function of body systems and tissues—in search of a better understanding of health and disease during and following pregnancy. Most physicians are ill informed or just plain ignorant when it comes to nutrition. This makes little sense, considering that every tissue in the body is made from the nutrients that come from what we eat and drink. The proteins, fats, carbohydrates, minerals, enzymes, and water we take in are the stuff that forms our bodies. Bones are made of protein and minerals. Muscles are mostly made up of protein, iron, vitamin B$_{12}$, and folic acid. The brain is composed of very specific fats and proteins. The structure and function of every organ, gland, muscle, and bone in our bodies are dependent upon adequate nutrition. When nutrient reserves are drawn upon heavily, or if nutritional intake is lacking in quality or quantity, the systems that keep the body running smoothly are affected at their most basic cellular levels. Various symptoms appear, depending on which body systems are not getting the nutrients they need.

A baby's body is built entirely from the nutrient reserves of its mother. If a developing baby is in need of key nutrients when there are not enough to go around, the baby's needs always come first. The mother is the one who goes without. As a result, any nutritional deficiencies affect the mother, and she is the one who suffers from health problems related to the lack of those nutrients. Of course, severe nutrient deficiencies can also affect her baby's development and health.

Many of the women we counsel about postpregnancy ailments insist that they ate better than they had ever eaten in their lives during and after their pregnancies, carefully calculating serving sizes and including plenty of protein, vegetables, and fruit. Most women also used prenatal vitamins. These women found it hard to believe that they could still be lacking in nutrients. However, while most prenatal vitamins have enough of the basic vitamins and minerals to fulfill the needs of the growing baby, they fall short of supplying adequate amounts for both baby and mother. In addition, some of the most crucial nutrient building blocks for the baby's body are completely missing from many prenatal vitamins. These nutrients, which will be discussed in detail in Chapter 7, are depleted from a pregnant woman's body at a high rate if she is not eating an abundance of the foods that supply them.

Conventional wisdom tells women that they no longer need to take vitamins after having their babies, although their bodies are probably more depleted than ever after the trials of labor. This is especially true if a woman lost a significant amount of blood during delivery or had to have an emergency C-section.

Joan's Story

Joan had been told by her obstetrician that vitamins would do nothing but give her "expensive urine," and he insisted that she should be able to get all of her nutrients from food. When Joan came to my office, she was three months pregnant, fatigued and depressed, and she got dizzy when she stood up quickly. She was extremely pale and had dark purplish circles under her eyes. Her blood pressure was low, and it fell further when she stood up from a lying-down position.

I measured Joan's iron, vitamin B_{12}, and folic-acid levels using a blood test known as a *chem* (short for chemistry) *screen*. Her levels of all three nutrients were low enough to be considered dangerous to her health and to the health of her baby—certainly low enough to explain all of her symptoms. I sent Joan on her way with supplements to raise her nutrient levels.

A few days later, Joan was back with questions. Her obstetrician/ gynecologist (OB/GYN) had scared her out of taking the supplements. He seemed offended that Joan had asked anyone else for advice. He had told her to drink a can of one of those so-called nutritional foods if she was concerned about her nutrient levels. Joan was confused. I explained to her that those "nutritional foods" are really mostly corn syrup and artificial flavoring, with a few chemical versions of vitamins mixed in— hardly a nutritionist's idea of good prenatal care! I also told Joan that low folic-acid levels in her baby's body could lead to birth defects such as spina bifida or cleft palate. Joan compromised by taking much lower doses of nutrients than I had prescribed. Fortunately, she had a healthy baby. When I saw her a few months later, however, she still looked pallid and complained of feeling "so tired." She had taken enough of the nutrients to help her baby but not enough to replenish her own reserves.

Later in this book, you will learn more about how vitamin B_{12}, folic acid, and iron deficiencies can cause subtle and not-so-subtle changes in energy and overall health.

—D.R.

The Problem of Postpartum Depression

During your pregnancy, you knew from your reading to expect emotional changes, but now you may be overwhelmed by worry and sadness. Where is the happiness you know you should be feeling? The fact that it seems beyond your grasp makes you feel even worse.

Despite being exhausted from the responsibilities of new motherhood, you lie awake at night worrying about your baby's health and your ability to mother him or her. During the day, you are constantly anxious about harm befalling your baby. You can barely think clearly enough to decide what to have for lunch, and the idea of making any kind of important decision about how to deal with issues that come up for your baby is more than you can stand. You realize that you must be suffering from postpartum depression.

Nearly every book on pregnancy and childbirth warns new mothers of the possibility of postpartum depression (PPD). In order to be diagnosed with PPD, you must suffer from depression, or lack interest in life, for most of the day, every day, for two weeks or more following the birth of a child. An estimated one new mother in ten experiences PPD. The level of depression may be constant, or it may be mild on some days and severe on others.

A diagnosis of PPD is not made unless at least four of the following symptoms are present:

- Changes in appetite or sleep patterns.
- Difficulty concentrating and making decisions.
- Excessive anxiety.
- Fatigue.
- Feelings of guilt or worthlessness; doubting your own ability to mother or feeling as though you are already a failure at it.
- Recurrent thoughts of death or suicide.
- Restlessness or lethargy.

While it seems likely that many of these symptoms would be commonplace in sleep-deprived women with new babies and bodies on the mend, they can become debilitating in a mother with PPD.

Postpartum depression is often confused with a milder, more fleeting, and more common form of depression known as the "baby blues." From half to three-quarters of all new moms get the blues in the first few days after giving birth. They may burst into tears for no apparent reason or be restless, irritable, and impatient (not so uncalled-for if you are dealing with a crying newborn and stitches in your most sensitive areas). This usually goes away on its own and is often attributed to the psychological letdown after the emotional high of giving birth. However, in many instances, the baby blues or a mild form of depression called dysthymia can be prolonged for months or even years postpartum if nutrient reserves are not replenished.

About one in every thousand women experiences postpartum psychosis, complete with hallucinations, delusions, severe insomnia, agitation, and bizarre behaviors. Rarely, women suffer from postpartum anxiety/panic disorder, which shows up as intense fear, rapid breathing and heart rate, hot or cold flashes, trembling, dizziness, and even chest pain. Postpartum obsessive-compulsive disorder (OCD) can also occur, although it too is rare. It is more likely to occur in women who have had OCD in the past.

A study of more than 35,000 women showed a sevenfold increase in the likelihood of being hospitalized with a psychiatric illness during the first three months postpartum. Of the approximately 11.4 million women who give birth each year in the United States, it is thought that about 40 percent have to work their way through some sort of mood disorder after giving birth.

Psychiatrists make distinctions among numerous forms of depression. *Unipolar* or *major depression* is a very serious form of depression, as is *bipolar disorder,* which is characterized by severe mood swings. We do not at all suggest that those with these more serious forms of depression depend solely on the nutrients suggested in this book. It is absolutely essential a person with a serious form of depression be under the care of a competent psychiatrist. We do look forward to the day that many more physicians will be educated in the use of the nutritional precursors to the brain neurotransmitters to help support such people nutritionally in addition to using pharmaceutical antidepressants.

Dysthymia, the more mild form of depression mentioned above, affects tens of millions of people, most of them women. Many of those who suffer from dysthymia can be helped by using nutraceuticals (nutrients taken in therapeutic dosages), either alone or as an adjunct to antidepressant drugs. The key here is to know that antidepressant drugs actually *deplete* the nutritional precursors the brain needs to make its own neurotransmitters and to find a physician experienced in the use of both nutritional and pharmaceutical protocols.

WHAT CAUSES POSTPARTUM DEPRESSION?

Women who have been depressed in the past are more likely to end up with PPD, and women who have had PPD with previous pregnancies have a 70 percent chance of having it again. Those with marital problems, abusive spouses, substance abuse problems, or a lack of social support are more likely to have PPD. Many experts feel that these factors are enough to explain the PPD phenomenon.

Other researchers believe that there is a biological mechanism at work. Fluctuations in hormones, including thyroid hormone, cortisol, prolactin, progesterone, and estrogen, can strongly influence a woman's emotional state. (We will address each of these hormones in greater detail in later chapters.) There is nothing like the transition from late-term pregnancy to new motherhood to toss one's hormones into complete disarray. Changes in brain levels of the neurotransmitters serotonin and norepinephrine also take place soon after a woman gives birth, and these changes are thought to be very important contributors to PPD as well. Deficiencies of the amino acids, vitamins, and minerals that form these neurotransmitters can severely limit the ability of the brain and nervous system to make them. We will discuss this in more detail in later chapters.

The scientific consensus is that PPD is multifactorial, which means that all of the above variables—hormonal, psychological, and neurochemical—come into play. We believe that all of these factors share one important and commonly overlooked characteristic: The balance of each of these systems relies upon proper nutrition. If the nutritional building blocks that the body needs to make hormones, neurotransmitters, and other mood-altering body chemicals are not present in adequate amounts, mood and physical health can both be compromised.

MEDICAL TREATMENT FOR POSTPARTUM DEPRESSION

As is the case with depression unrelated to pregnancy, mood-altering drugs and psychotherapy are conventional medicine's treatments of choice for PPD. While talking to a trusted friend or psychotherapist is often helpful, the usefulness of the drugs most often prescribed for women with PPD has not yet been proven. Most physicians treat PPD with various psychiatric drugs that, in effect, trick the brain into thinking it has more neurotransmitters than it actually does—specifically, that levels of one or both of two very important brain neurotransmitters, serotonin and nor-epinephrine, have been increased. Serotonin and norepinephrine are fundamental to a healthy body because they carry nerve signals and messages throughout the brain and the rest of the nervous system. They have a profound effect on mood and self-esteem, as well as on many other important functions within the body. A deficiency of these neurotransmitters can lead to depression, anxiety, insomnia, anger, obesity, and a host of other serious ailments.

In the vast majority of cases of PPD, the real cause of low levels of serotonin or norepinephrine in the brain is a deficiency of the nutritional precursors that the body needs to make these neurotransmitters. Interestingly, not only do the psychiatric drugs most commonly prescribed for PPD *not* increase serotonin and neroepinephrine levels, but they actually cause the body's reserves of the nutritional precursors needed to produce them to be used up more rapidly, worsening the state of nutritional deficiency. This is probably why it is so difficult for so many people to go off these drugs. It is not unusual for doctors to hear that a person had a very good initial experience with one of these drugs but that, as time passed, the good feelings wore off and higher doses and/or different medications were needed.

The most common class of drugs physicians prescribe for PPD is known as selective serotonin reuptake inhibitors, or SSRIs, the best-known of which is fluoxetine (Prozac). Other medications in this category include citalopram (Celexa), paroxetine (Paxil), and sertraline (Zoloft). These agents act by keeping serotonin in the brain's synapses (the spaces between nerve cells) for a longer period of time. They also pull serotonin out of the "serotonin stores" in the brain cells and pull it into the synapses. However, as we learn so tragically from time to time when we hear of mothers on medication for PPD who harm or even kill their children, these drugs don't always work. In fact, they fail to work over the long term at least one-third of the time. SSRIs speed up the rate at which serotonin is used up in the brain. If you drive a car at a high rate of speed, it uses up more gas and you have to fill up the tank more often. Similarly, if you speed up the rate at which the brain uses up serotonin by taking SSRIs you will need to replace the nutritional precursors more rapidly.

Why are so many people apparently suffering the effects of low serotonin levels? There are a number of reasons. Serotonin and a group of neurotransmitters called the catecholamines—adrenaline (epinephrine), noradrenaline (norepinephrine), and dopamine—which are predominantly made by the adrenal glands, work together and need to be in balance within the nervous system. As the general level of stress with which we live has gone up, our adrenal glands have been induced to make more catecholamines. The brain then is faced with the need to make more serotonin to maintain a proper balance. It is estimated that the level of stress most of us face on a daily basis is 100 times higher than that faced by our grandparents. The world keeps getting more complicated, and our nervous systems keep trying to adapt. We have reached a point at which many people's brains are having trouble making enough serotonin to match the levels of adrenal catecholamines required to cope with life.

There are a number of other factors that make it more difficult for our brains to produce enough serotonin. The brain needs a steady supply of the amino acid tryptophan and vitamin B_6 to make serotonin. Proteins in foods contain a very small percentage of tryptophan as compared with other amino acids. Only about 3 percent of the tryptophan in food is actually converted into serotonin in the brain. This is partly due to the fact that about 95 percent of the serotonin in the body is needed and used in the intestinal tract. Further, to reach the brain, tryptophan must be ferried across the blood-brain barrier (a protective mechanism in the brain that keeps certain substances from easily entering the inner sanctum of the brain) by means of a carrier protein. Tryptophan has to compete with other amino acids for these carrier proteins, and this limits the amount of tryptophan that can enter the brain at any given time. Further, the adrenal hormone cortisol, which is produced in response to stress, converts tryptophan into a chemical called *kynurenine,* which cannot be converted into serotonin. If you drink coffee, smoke cigarettes, drink alcohol, eat chocolate, take diet pills, or just have a lot of stress in your life—and what mother doesn't?— your body will produce too much cortisol, increasing the amount of tryptophan that is converted to kynurenine and limiting the amount available to produce serotonin.

To make matters even a bit more difficult, the production of serotonin does not take place in a single step, but is a complicated biochemical process, and each of the steps along the way requires specific nutrients. Your body must have enough iron and vitamin B_3 (niacin) to convert tryptophan into a compound known as 5-hydroxy-L-tryptophan (5-HTP) *and* enough other B vitamins plus the mineral magnesium to convert vitamin B_6 to pyridoxal-5-phosphate (P5P), the form necessary for serotonin production. Without enough 5-HTP and P5P available in the brain, serotonin cannot be made at adequate levels. Doctors cannot simply give their patients serotonin orally or intravenously because serotonin is fat soluble and does not pass through the blood-brain barrier. The only way that the brain can get serotonin is to make it from the specific nutritional precursors available to it at the time. (Fortunately, 5-HTP and P5P are available in supplement form; more about this in Chapter 7.)

All of these factors can lead to an individual having an inadequate supply of serotonin for optimal health, and in turn may explain the startling statistic that an estimated one in ten Americans—and one in four women!—is now on SSRI drugs.

The safety of SSRIs for the babies of nursing mothers also has not been proven. Some studies have linked the maternal use of Prozac to colic in nursing infants. A baby with colic can push the most even-tempered mother over the edge. For this reason alone, giving such a drug to a mom with PPD doesn't seem like the best way to support her recovery. Further, Prozac and similar drugs pass into a nursing mother's milk and, thus, into her baby's body. While studies have shown that little or no drug circulates in a baby's bloodstream, others that have looked at the concentrations of the drug in babies' brain tissue have found much higher levels. Nothing is known about the possible harm this can do to a newborn.

Some mothers choose to take the drugs and not to nurse. This deprives their babies of the most perfect food they can be given, and deprives both mother and child of the important bonding that comes with breast-feeding. Mothers with PPD who miss out on the bonding experience of breastfeeding may end up feeling even more distant from their babies. Most of the mothers we have consulted with who chose to take SSRIs over breastfeeding would have chosen to nurse if they had felt there was any other way to heal PPD. Unfortunately, mainstream medicine routinely tells new mothers with PPD that these drugs are the only way out.

The dangers of SSRIs go beyond their dangers to the baby. One potential side effect of these drugs is a feeling of numbness, of separateness from others. Feeling numb does tend to blunt depression, but it may do so at the expense of a new mother's feelings of intimacy with her baby and her partner at this crucial time. The most common side effects of SSRIs include nausea, sleepiness, insomnia, sexual dysfunction, headaches, trembling, indigestion, abdominal pain, and nervousness. SSRI drugs also seem to lift normal inhibitions against violence and suicide in some people. Prozac has been linked with violence toward others, suicide, and self-mutilation, and thus may even play a part in enabling an over-wrought woman to commit one of the worst crimes imaginable—causing serious harm to her child. Many experts, including Harvard University psychiatrist and author Joseph Glenmullen, M.D., and Peter R. Breggin, M.D., psychiatrist, author, and director of the nonprofit International Center for the Study of Psychiatry and Psychology (ICSPP), warn that SSRIs are overprescribed and that their dangers are drastically under-played.

Dr. Glenmullen's most recent book, *Prozac Backlash* (Simon & Schuster, 2000), warns that SSRIs can cause symptoms similar to those of Parkinson's disease—including facial and body tics and muscle spasms that may persist even after the drug is discontinued—in at least 10 percent of those who use them. This finding implies that SSRIs may create dangerously low levels of the neurotransmitter dopamine in some people. Moreover, the long-term effects of Prozac and similar drugs are not known, but some studies indicate that permanent brain damage could occur because the constant artificial elevation of the neurotransmitter serotonin eventually burns out the serotonin receptor sites in the brain and makes them unable to respond.

The manufacturer of Prozac insists that no link between the drug and suicide has been proven. Interestingly, however, they will be marketing a newer version of the antidepressant, which, according to published reports, they will advertise as less likely to cause suicide and violent behavior in those who use it—raising the question of why they would use this issue as a selling point. The "new Prozac," R-fluoxetine, is set to hit the market just as the patent for the current version, which has had sales in excess of $2 billion a year, runs out. Incidentally, Sarafem, an antidepressant that is being marketed heavily for a form of premenstrual syndrome (PMS), is chemically identical to Prozac—with a different, female consumer–savvy name.

Serotonin does seem to play a role in depression, and that is why SSRIs can provide relief. Keep in mind, however, that no one has shown that a chemical imbalance—in this case, low serotonin levels—is the sole cause of depression. Boosting serotonin will improve most people's moods, but this symptomatic relief at best because the nutritional precursors the brain needs to produce its own serotonin remain depleted unless deliberately replenished. As Dr. Breggin says in his book *Talking Back to Prozac* (St. Martin's Press, 1994), depression is not caused by a Prozac deficiency any more than a headache is caused by an aspirin deficiency.

Fortunately for those who wish to avoid SSRIs, there are ways to elevate serotonin levels naturally with foods and supplements. (You will find out how in Chapters 5 and 7.) We believe that taking SSRIs can make things worse for many women who suffer from PPD, and we do not recommend using them, especially over the long term, unless you have one of the more serious forms of depression. If you do need them for the short term, you should enlist your doctor's assistance to help you wean yourself off them as soon as possible. Never stop using SSRIs abruptly, however, as this can cause serious withdrawal symptoms. Taper off gradually with the guidance of a knowledgeable physician, preferably one who is experienced in prescribing increasing amounts of the nutritional precursors you need as you wean off the drugs.

Many women suffer from a kind of depression that results not at all from low brain serotonin levels but from low levels of another brain neurotransmitter, norepinephrine. Increasing serotonin levels with drugs does not help this kind of depression. On the contrary, it often makes people even more tired and depressed. Women with low serotonin levels tend to have a great deal of anxiety, while women with low norepinephrine levels feel like they fell into a deep, dark hole and just cannot muster the energy to get out of it, or elicit more than one positive thought in a row. People with low norepinephrine levels are often dramatically helped by restoring normal thyroid and adrenal gland function. The amino acid tyrosine, along with P5P, copper, iron, and vitamin C, is necessary to make norepinephrine. Tyrosine, along with the mineral iodine, is also the main nutritional precursor for all the thyroid hormones. (This will be discussed in Chapter 9.)

As you will discover as you move through this book, we believe that the vast majority of cases of PPD can be prevented and/or treated very successfully without resorting to drugs that may harm you and your baby. The natural strategies presented in this book can help to restore serotonin levels and replenish key nutrients and other biochemicals that are likely to be depleted as a result of bringing a child into the world. In the chapters that follow, we will see how a woman's nutritional status is affected by pregnancy and birth, how this can determine her overall state of health, and, most important, what she can do to regain a state of balance and well-being.

2

Pregnancy Preparation,
Support, and Recovery

If a conventional medical doctor were to glance at this book, he or she might think, "What's this 'pregnancy recovery' thing about? Women have been having babies for millions of years, giving birth and going back to their work. Suddenly women need instructions on how to recover from pregnancy?"

Legend tells of the hardy tribeswoman who can squat down in the fields, push her baby out, strap it to her back, and keep right on plowing. While we can't say that this never happens, we can say that you certainly should not expect the same of yourself. Legends are about exceptions, not norms. To remain healthy on a long-term basis, every woman should have some rest and recovery time after giving birth. We're sure that this mythical tribeswoman would appreciate it if someone else took over the plowing and let her spend a few days resting after the birth of her child. Considering that the average life expectancy of such a woman would be about thirty-five years, we suspect this type of lifestyle is hard on her!

It used to be that a woman who had a baby in a hospital got a break of at least a few days, but in this era of managed health care, the length of time she can spend recovering in the hospital has been steadily decreasing. In the 1960s and 1970s, most new mothers stayed in the hospital with their newborns for five days to a week. In the 1950s, the usual hospital stay after childbirth was closer to two weeks. A few years ago, a new mother could leave after forty-eight hours, providing she had a normal vaginal birth. This was because it would take this long to make sure that the baby had no health problems; the mother's opportunity to stay in bed for a couple of days and do nothing but bond with her baby and be waited on hand and foot was a fringe benefit.

Today, if mother and child are deemed to be basically healthy, they are encouraged to go home only hours after the birth. Again, this is not for the benefit of the mother—or for the baby. It is for the benefit of managed health-care organizations that pinch every penny they spend on behalf of their clients even as they pay their top executives yearly salaries high enough to erase the national debts of small Third World countries.

While many women are glad to leave the hospital as soon as possible after the birth of a child, it can be difficult to take the time to recuperate once you get home. There may be other children who need to be cared for, meals may need to be prepared, the house may need to be cleaned. Some moms feel that they are expected to jump right back into the fray without missing a step.

Pregnancy Recovery (or the Lack Thereof) Then and Now

A hundred years ago, women would stay in bed for a couple of weeks after giving birth to recover their strength and to bond with the new baby. Even today, traditional home birth midwives tell new mothers to stay in bed for two weeks, getting up only to go to the bathroom and to eat. Such practitioners visit mothers at home three or four times in the postpartum weeks to check on the baby and to sit and talk with the mother about her birth experience, her feelings about the baby, her own physical complaints, or whatever other issues arise. If the baby or mother needs medical care for minor problems, they need not get in the car and go to a doctor's office; the home-birth midwife comes to them. Many midwives place a sign on the door of the mother's home, instructing visitors to keep visits short during the first weeks of the baby's life and to pitch in with chores and food preparation while they are there.

Bed rest is also a mainstay of postpartum recovery in traditional Chinese medicine. For centuries, new mothers in many parts of China have been encouraged to eat a soup made from the placenta that is cooked very, very slowly over the lowest possible heat. This practice has been followed in many cultures, over many centuries, all over the world. The concept of eating the placenta may be unappetizing to Westerners, but it is a powerful way to immediately begin to replenish nutritional deficiencies and depletions after giving birth. Many mammals eat the placenta, and this could very well be the reason they do not need much down time after giving birth. The placenta is rich in protein, iron, folic acid, vitamin B_{12}, vitamin B_6, and hormones such as progesterone. The progesterone the placenta contains probably helps bring the body back into hormonal balance. (In Chapter 9, we will explore how the steep postpartum drop in progesterone contributes to postpartum ailments.)

Obviously, few modern women would choose to eat the placenta, so they need to pay special attention to providing their bodies with similarly nourishing foods and supplements postpartum. Traditional Chinese postpartum care also includes a fish soup containing *san qi (Panax notoginseng),* an herb known in the West as *pseudoginseng*. You might consider doing the same if your health practitioner feels that pseudoginseng is appropriate for you. This soup supplies the body with proteins, vitamins, and minerals. (A recipe for fish soup with seaweed appears in Chapter 5.)

Many other approaches to the process of preparing for, supporting the body during, and recovering from childbirth exist throughout the world today. There is plenty of wisdom from both ancient cultures and the most modern alternative medicine to help American mothers (who arguably have the least support after pregnancy than women in any other developed nation) recover from the stress and strain of pregnancy and childbirth.

To give you a better grasp of some of the advice you will find throughout the rest of this book, we will now share some of the basics about how a number of the healing practices we use can mix and match in the way we treat our patients. These practices include traditional Chinese medicine, functional medicine, chiropractic, applied kinesiology, and the use of modern research–based plant medicines. Understanding these approaches will give you the understanding to apply the advice in chapters to come.

TRADITIONAL CHINESE MEDICINE:
ANCIENT PRACTICES, MODERN USES

The theories and practices of traditional Chinese medicine (TCM) have been around for five millennia, and they are still used today in the health care of a large percentage of the world's population. In TCM, health is a complex, ever-shifting balance of subtle energy called *qi* (pronounced "chee," sometimes spelled *chi*) that interweaves body, mind, and environment. TCM does not necessarily view declining health as an indication that some foreign element called disease has invaded the body; rather, it shows that the body's energy has become unbalanced and must be gently guided back to its balance point. One key element of this concept is that the health of all living things is dependent on the balanced flow of electromagnetic energy nourishing all the tissues of the body. Ideally, this life-sustaining electromagnetic energy moves freely through invisible vessels or channels called meridians. These acupuncture meridians function much as blood vessels do in that they help guide the movement of qi so it can provide the needed flow of electrons to each tissue and cell in the body. If the qi is imbalanced within a person and between the person and her environment, disease is the eventual result.

Every person has her own ideal balance point, at which she feels healthiest. If the body cannot make the shift back to that point, imbalance results. This can manifest itself in subtle or not-so-subtle ways—as weakened immunity, allergies, yeast infections, fatigue, pain, emotional imbalances, or other ailments. The TCM practitioner gently aids the body in coming back into balance. Herbs, special foods, needle protocols (that is, acupuncture), and supplements boost the body's resistance to disease and ability to heal. Acupuncture, in which hair-fine needles are used to stimulate specific points along the body's meridians, restores the flow of qi, helping to move healing energy through the body.

With the development of functional medicine and clinical nutrition over the past half-century, a perfect modern complement to these ancient practices now exists.

FUNCTIONAL MEDICINE: YOU ARE WHAT YOU EAT

Why is it that when you catch a cold, your spouse or children are often spared? Because you are more stressed, depleted, and deprived of sleep than anyone else in the house. You may have been living on pizza and macaroni and cheese because that is all you have the energy to make, and you have probably been devoting most of your waking moments to caring for an infant. Your immune system doesn't get its fair share of resources when you are in this state, and so it cannot prevent the cold virus from knocking you flat. A TCM practitioner might describe this imbalance as follows: The lifestyle of the typical new mother disrupts the balance of energy in her body, which makes her body more vulnerable to illness.

Functional medicine is a sort of super-modern complement to TCM that looks deeply into the way each person's body takes in food, breaks it down, uses it to make energy, and disposes of waste. TCM is all about energy balance between body systems, and functional medicine addresses the cellular processes that make energy in each and every living cell as well as the whole body system.

Complex microscopic systems in the cells transform proteins, carbohydrates, and fats to energy; other systems apply that energy to the work of each cell. Vitamins, minerals, and other nutrients from food are the cogs, wheels, and sparks that make these tiny engines run. (In Chapter 3, you will learn more about how these systems work and about the indispensable roles that nutrients from foods play in them.) The more we unravel the mysteries of genetics and of how genes interact with the environment, the more we recognize that there are subtle but important differences in the way each person's body goes about these processes.

Your body's unique genetic makeup and its interaction with the environment you live in—what Jeffrey Bland, Ph.D., one of functional medicine's champions, refers to as your "life context"—translates to a unique set of nutritional needs. Those needs can change over time, especially during the course of pregnancy, birth, and early motherhood.

According to this approach, you can have a dysfunction that is unique to you and that does not necessarily manifest itself as full-blown disease. This might show up as a group of vague complaints, such as fatigue, mood changes, achiness, or gastrointestinal discomforts. All too often, people are told that, because their complaints do not fit into the conventional medical diagnostic framework, there is really nothing wrong with them—despite the fact that they feel awful. In functional medicine, we don't wait until you fall into the conventional category of "sick" before we try to help you feel better. We remedy dysfunction as soon as it is noticeable.

Like TCM and chiropractic, functional medicine seeks to treat the root of the problem rather than the symptoms. Its main tool is nutrition—supplying the body with the nutrients it needs to attain its healthiest balance. This approach works especially well with postpregnancy ailments that develop out of the nutrient drain of pregnancy and birthing. There are functional medicine laboratory tests performed by nationally accredited labs that can measure specific deficiencies in key nutrients such as fatty acids, amino acids, minerals, organic acids, and many other important nutrients necessary to run the body's metabolic pathways.

CHIROPRACTIC CARE: MUCH MORE THAN BACK-CRACKING

Chiropractic has been a distinct health-care practice since 1895, but its underlying tenets have been applied by healers since ancient Greek times. The chiropractic approach may have begun with Hippocrates, the Greek physician who is considered the father of modern medicine, when he said, "Whatever the problem, first look to the spine."

The focus of chiropractic is on the proper alignment of the *vertebrae,* the bones that make up the spine. The transmission of information from the brain throughout the body and back to the brain all happens through the spinal cord. Chiropractic views the spinal cord literally as an elongation of the brain that allows communication with the muscles, organs, glands, and other tissues of the body through the nerves that branch from it. You can think of the brain as the generator and the spine as the main power line, with smaller power lines branching off to bring nervous system energy to where it is needed. If anything disrupts the integrity of those power lines, the energy flow is going to be disrupted as well.

The stacked vertebrae that make up the spinal column form a protective passageway for the spinal cord. Openings between the vertebrae allow nerves to branch off the cord to the organs, muscles, and skin. Information cannot move through the nervous system properly if the bones that encase the spinal cord and the nerves that branch off of it are out of place. Displaced, or *subluxated,* vertebrae can have profound effects on organ function, joint stability, muscles, and posture. A subluxated vertebra can cause too much or too little energy to be transmitted to muscles and organs. While this will not necessarily manifest itself immediately as a serious health problem, it can be compared to static coming through on your radio rather than a clear signal. Over time, the lack of clarity in the messages sent back and forth via the nervous system can cause problems. While subluxations can cause pain, muscle or organ problems can exist even if there is no pain. A skilled chiropractor can identify and "adjust" spinal subluxations, reestablishing proper alignment.

Carrying the weight of a six- to eight-pound baby in your belly, plus the extra pounds of pregnancy, places a lot of stress on the spine—not to mention the havoc the work of childbirth can wreak on the alignment of the vertebrae and the pelvis. After giving birth, you spend much of your time lifting and toting your baby in your arms, or assuming the head-forward position of nursing. Many postpartum women can benefit from chiropractic adjustments.

APPLIED KINESIOLOGY

The practice of applied kinesiology entails a series of muscle tests, based on an evaluation of a person's posture, that allows the doctor to accurately determine which muscles are not functioning well and why.

If specific muscles are weakened, they become unable to adequately stabilize and mobilize joints. Weak muscles make the body more vulnerable to injury, limit one's ability to move properly, and can cause muscle and joint pain or even joint subluxations. Applied kinesiology identifies these weaknesses and allows the practitioner to find and correct the cause of the weak muscles.

Muscular weaknesses can tell a skilled practitioner more about your body than you might think. One of the great contributions of applied kinesiology is the awareness that specific muscles share the same "nerve circuit" as specific organs or glands. These muscle/organ circuits are called *viscerosomatic reflexes,* and are hardwired into the spinal cord. The muscle-testing techniques of applied kinesiology help the practitioner to determine whether a muscle is weak because of a problem with the nerves that connect it to the central nervous system; a problem with its supply of blood, lymph, or nutrients; or an imbalance in the acupuncture meridian that supplies electromagnetic energy to the muscle. Sometimes, the problem can be traced back to the organ that shares the same circuit. Muscles can even be "turned off," or inhibited, by unresolved emotional issues. Various techniques have been developed to restore proper function to weakened muscles within the practice of applied kinesiology.

Think of this relationship between muscles and organs as a circuit breaker in a house. When a circuit is overloaded and the breaker is tripped, the appliances to which it feeds power stop working. Energy pathways in the body work the same way. When the organs are stressed, the nerve input overloads the circuit and the muscles along that circuit "turn off." Acupuncture, herbs, adjustments that realign structure, specific nutrients, and *chi kung* (specific exercises designed to alter the energy flow in the body) are used to replenish the organs and turn those energy circuits back on.

Applied kinesiology expands the concepts of chiropractic to take into consideration the alignment of the cranial (skull) bones, the temporo-mandibular joint (TMJ; the hinge that joins the jaw to the skull), and all of the extremities, including the hips, knees, ankles, feet, shoulders, elbows, wrists, and hands. A well-trained, board-certified applied kinesiologist (a diplomate of the International Board of Applied Kinesiology, or DIBAK) can often help you discover the cause of functional health problems—the kinds of problems that stump the average physician. Only licensed doctors of the various healing arts—doctors of chiropractic (D.C.s), medical doctors (M.D.s), doctors of osteopathy (D.O.s), and doctors of dentistry (DDSs)—can earn this certification, after undertaking at least three years of study and passing certifying examinations.

Chiropractic—specifically, applied kinesiology—can be helpful not only to a mother during pregnancy and postpartum, but to the baby as well. We favor using applied kinesiology techniques to adjust expectant mothers every few weeks during pregnancy, and to gently align both mother and baby soon after birth. The cranium of a baby delivered vaginally must withstand tremendous pressure during the process of being born. A well-trained and experienced cranial expert can gently restore proper cranial alignment soon after birth so that the baby's head forms properly and, more important, the baby's brain functions optimally.

PLANT MEDICINES

We humans have probably been using plants medicinally for as long as we have been on earth. In fact, even animals instinctively eat medicinal plants when they need them. The majority of the world's cultures still use plants as their primary medicines. Plant medicines fell into disrepute in the United States with the advent of synthetic medicines—substances not found in nature, though often based on compounds originally extracted from plants—that could be patented and that therefore were highly profitable. Drug companies and conventional medicine campaigned fiercely against plant medicines during the twentieth century, claiming that they were not safe or effective, and that their use was not based on science. This negative campaign was based not so much on truth as on economic incentives and a desire to eliminate competition. While some synthetic pharmaceutical drugs, such as antibiotics and certain painkillers, have clearly had a profound and positive impact on the health and well-being of humanity, the majority of them can do as much harm as good because of harsh side effects. Deaths in hospitals alone from *correctly prescribed* prescription drugs are among the top ten causes of death in the United States. Deaths attributed to properly used plant medicines are virtually nonexistent, even in cultures where they are widely used.

In the past few decades there has been a huge grassroots movement in the United States back toward the more gentle plant medicines, along with a trend toward treating health problems with nutritional supplements. Scientific research on the constituents and effects of plant medicines has boomed in the past twenty years. In most cases, science has found that the active components of plant medicines have identifiable effects on the human body that match the plants' use in folk medicine. Plant medicines are widely used in many parts of Europe, and German scientists in particular have extensively researched the constituents and effects of herbal medicines. For many conditions, German physicians are as likely to write prescriptions for plant medicines as for pharmaceutical drugs.

While we both recommend pharmaceutical drugs when we perceive that they are needed, most of the medicinal treatments we recommend come from plants or specific nutrients. We have found that this approach creates the most trouble-free short-term healing, as well as the most effective long-term healing.

Moving In and Out of Health

Sometimes, the cause-and-effect relationship of an illness is obvious: an infection of the nasal passages by a certain strain of virus causes the symptoms of the common cold; bacteria multiplying in the milk ducts causes the painful inflammation of mastitis. With many other common postpartum complaints, however, the relationship is not so simple. Women who suffer from deep fatigue, sadness, irritability, gastrointestinal problems, skin rashes, headaches, or worsening of allergies or asthma postpartum are usually told by their doctors that the cause of their discomfort is a mystery—and that the only option is to use potent drugs to treat symptoms. The use of prescription drugs often makes underlying nutrient deficiencies worse. As you will see in Chapter 3, nutrients are needed to utilize and to detoxify these drugs. Those nutrients come from the body's stores, depleting those stores all the more quickly.

Many of the patients we see have already been to conventional doctors, who have explained that there is nothing really *wrong* with them because their symptoms do not fit the conventional framework. If symptoms cannot be classified, diagnosed as a disease, and treated with medicines, they are not sick. Still, these women know they are not functioning optimally. If this is a good description of your own plight, you should find answers in these pages.

We don't try to put our patients into categories of "sick" or "not sick." When we see a patient, we look at her past history and present symptoms, and get a sense of where that particular person's ideal state of health is. We compare that to where she is now, and we try to make the adjustments that will bring her back to that ideal place. It usually takes more time and more attention than diagnosing a "Prozac deficiency," but this approach is a real cure for the problem instead of a pharmaceutical Band-Aid. Why just turn off the fire alarm when you can actually put out the fire?

No two people—not even identical twins—require exactly the same interventions. Even identical twin women marry different men, live in different households, have different jobs, eat different diets, and experience different kinds of stress. That said, there are certain guidelines we use as clinicians to help us see whether someone is moving out of health in a general sense. More detailed diagnostic methods help us to home in on specific problems.

If you were to walk into either of our offices, we would start with an evaluation of your appearance. We would look at your posture and at the vibrancy of your skin. What kind of energy did you have as you entered the room? Do you have a generally tired look? Did you slump into the chair, or do you seem jumpy or irritable? All of this is important information.

Sometimes a woman comes into the office looking as though she is completely exhausted, with pale, sallow skin and tensed shoulders, and when she is asked if she feels tired or anxious, she says no. So many women push themselves so hard toward goals and tasks, toward getting things done, that they have in effect dissociated themselves from their bodies. They come to see us about a specific ailment that has become too serious to ignore, but they really do not feel how exhausted they are. Many shrug off their exhaustion as an unavoidable part of new motherhood, and it is true that new babies mean wakeful nights and trying days. Our job is to figure out whether our methods of improving functional reserves can give them a boost.

Most of the women who look exhausted but say that they are fine really know, deep down, that they could be feeling and functioning better than they are. Admitting that you are unwell and making the changes you need to make to move back into health can be difficult when you are trying to be Supermom, but the sooner you do so, the sooner you can get on the road to recovery. If you avoid the issue, your body will send you increasingly stern messages to take better care of yourself, and eventually you will not have a choice. If you wait that long, you will have a lot more work to do than if you had listened to the earlier, subtler signals.

At the initial office visit, we ask a lot of questions about when a patient's health problems started and about her experience of those problems. For example, we might ask whether the patient seems to catch every bug that comes through, and whether she finds that she heals slowly from injuries. We examine her tongue and the membranes in her nose and eyes. A tongue that looks as though it has a coating on it, or that has grooves or deep fissures in it, is evidence of specific nutritional problems. In people moving out of health, the membranes in the nose and eyes may be dried, cracked, and irritated.

We advocate measuring a woman's pulse, analyzing her posture, checking her whole structure for malalignments, and using applied kinesiology to help find the best healing solutions for her—performing a simple series of tests to measure the strength or weakness of muscle groups throughout the body. These tests yield important information that helps to diagnose and treat health problems. We order laboratory tests to measure nutrient and hormone levels, and other tests depending upon a patient's symptoms. The results of those tests help to show us how to proceed in bringing her individual system back to its own individual state of balance.

Laying the Foundations
of Pregnancy Recovery

Being in a state of health does not mean being completely free from physical and emotional discomfort. It is impossible to feel great 100 percent of the time, especially when you are enduring the stresses of pregnancy, birthing, and caring for a baby. A state of health is what allows you to meet these challenges with fortitude and flexibility. Vibrant good health allows you to weather the occasional cold or flu, the occasional period of sadness, or the more than occasional sleepless night without being knocked

Judy's Story

A few days after birthing a beautiful son, Judy developed a severe, pounding headache in her temples that worsened when she stood up. I found that her blood pressure dropped when she stood up from a seated position, which caused her to become lightheaded. Her neck and lower back were painful, especially near the sacroiliac joints in her pelvis.

A blood test revealed low total iron levels: 42 out of a possible range of 40 to 160. Her white blood cell count was also low, at 3,700, with a possible range of 4,000 to 10,000. Tests of immune function revealed that her white blood cell counts had fallen out of their proper balance. These findings pointed to deficiencies in the blood-building nutrients. Anemia, poor circulation, and lack of antioxidant nutrients all point to blood deficiency, and can be remedied with proper nutrition. Traditional Chinese practitioners called this a blood deficiency syndrome.

I performed chiropractic alignments and acupuncture. The chiropractic adjustments shifted Judy's pelvis and spine into their most balanced state, while acupuncture helped those adjustments to hold and to stimulate points that assist the body to more efficiently produce blood. Key pelvis-related muscles are on the same energy "circuit" as the adrenal glands. When the adrenals are overstressed, muscles that stabilize these joints are "turned off" and they become unstable. The B vitamins and vitamin C are essential for good adrenal function, and for someone like Judy, supplementing with them helps to get the adrenals going again, turn these muscles back on, and restabilize the pelvic joints.

Judy took liquid iron, vitamin B_{12}, and folic acid, as well as vitamin B_6, a multimineral supplement, pantothenic acid (sometimes referred to as vitamin B_5), Siberian ginseng, vitamin C, and glucosamine sulfate. It took about three weeks for these nutrients to begin to restore Judy's organs, muscles, and joints. Her back and neck pain were gone within three weeks. Her headaches diminished in a week's time and were completely gone within three weeks.

If these treatments had not worked, I would have gone on to give Judy an adrenal stress index test to determine whether her adrenals had become too exhausted to recover with only nutritional intervention. Sometimes, supplementary adrenal hormones such as DHEA or cortisol are needed along with vitamin and herbal support. (This will be discussed in Chapter 9.)

—D.R.

out of balance. It means not suffering from chronic conditions that never seem to go away and that keep you from enjoying your baby and your life. This is the kind of health we are promoting.

Physicians who practice medicine the way we do are becoming easier to find, but they are still few and far between. If you cannot find anyone in your town who will guide you back to health using the methods we describe in this book, never fear. While this book is no substitute for the care of a physician, it will help you to lay the foundation for a replenished, balanced body postpartum. It will also enable you to ask better questions when you do need professional medical care.

In chapters to come, you will find out how nutrient depletion during pregnancy and postpartum sets you up for chronic ailments. We will then give you the tools you need to prevent depletion or to remedy it if it is already affecting your health. We will give you guidelines to help you understand the results of lab tests and to read your own symptoms to find where you need extra nutritional or hormonal support. In subsequent chapters, you will learn the basics of restocking your nutrient reserves with food and supplements, and how to use natural hormones if you need them. Finally, we address some emotional and spiritual aspects of new motherhood that, when dealt with appropriately, can tip the scales back toward the balance of true good health—not only for the benefit of the new mom, but also for the benefit of her baby.

3

How Nutrient Depletion Sets the Stage for Postpartum Ailments

In this chapter, we will introduce you to some of the incredible goings-on within your body that keep you perking along day in and day out. *Functional nutrition* is about staying healthy by conscientiously supporting your body with the nutrients it needs to stay in tip-top working condition. This approach is similar to the periodic preventive maintenance you do on your car. By regularly changing the oil and checking all of the fluids, you help to prevent your car from breaking down. By identifying levels of nutrients that are getting low in your body and supplementing them, you do preventive maintenance against ill health.

A woman who has recently had a baby is like a car that has been driven from Vermont to San Francisco. That car is really going to need some maintenance by the time it rumbles across the Golden Gate Bridge. You wouldn't expect that car to run well for long if you simply kept putting gas in the gas tank and neglected the systems that combust that fuel, would you? You owe it to yourself (and your baby) to care for yourself at least as well as you would care for that car!

Making Informed Choices
about Your Health

The miraculous array of interior workings that keep your body going might appear to be complex at first glance, but beneath that complexity lies a beautiful simplicity. An understanding of the ways in which these body systems work paves the way for you to make the right choices in your quest to support them.

Let's go back to the car analogy for a moment more. Suppose that when you take your car to a repair shop, a mechanic you don't know well tells you that your car needs a lot of expensive work. Unless you are knowledgeable about the workings of cars, and of your own car in particular, you have to take the mechanic's word for it. You could easily end up paying big bucks for repairs you don't need. Possessing a basic understanding of how your body works—and developing a familiarity with your very own make and model—will help you create your own routine maintenance program and allow you to troubleshoot when something goes wrong. If you do need the aid of a health-care provider, you can make informed choices about the treatments he or she recommends.

For simplicity's sake, we have broken down the everyday workings of your body into four categories: *metabolism, detoxification, fat balance,* and *nervous-system balance*. These categories do not present a complete picture of everything that happens in your body, but in our experience, seeing patients day in and day out, these are the systems most powerfully affected by the nutrient depletion so often seen in new moms. The *endocrine,* or hormonal, system is also important—so important that we devote an entire chapter (Chapter 9) to the hormonal changes that occur during and after pregnancy. There is considerable overlap between all five of these systems; if any of them is not working up to par, the other four are strongly affected.

Healing Postpartum Ailments at the Functional Level

A nutrient deficiency of some sort is likely to occur in a woman who has just given up many of her reserves to make a baby's body. This nutrient lack can be compounded by not having as much rest and recovery time as her body requires after giving birth, and by not having the time or energy to take good care of herself because of the demands of her new baby.

Nutrient depletion does not always have obvious repercussions right away. If you are sick enough to go see a doctor, you can bet that your body started falling out of balance long before you made that appointment. Once you learn about how nutrients affect the most basic operations of your body, you will be better prepared to take steps to replenish them.

System 1: Metabolism— How Your Cells Make Energy

One of the most common postpartum symptoms is a lack of energy. While some fatigue is certainly par for the course, debilitating fatigue—such that day after day you feel you cannot even get out of bed—is not. Some women say they are absolutely exhausted and yet cannot sleep at night, even while their babies are sleeping. We have found that many women who lack energy also complain about weakness in their muscles and a rapid heart rate. The good news is that many women who thought their fatigue was normal have been surprised at how much more energetic they *can* be with a few nutritional and lifestyle adjustments.

Let's go down to the cellular level and examine what happens there to drain your energy reserves. This may sound complicated at first, but hang in there and you will discover why it is so important to get the right nutrients to maintain your energy.

Where does your body get energy from? You probably know that the food you eat is metabolized, or "burned," in your body to make energy. The foods you eat are broken down into their most basic components in your digestive system, or gastrointestinal tract. These basic nutrient components—*amino acids* from protein foods, *glucose* (sugar) from carbohydrates, and *fatty acids* from fats—are then absorbed into tiny blood and lymphatic vessels that line the intestines. The nutrients then either pass through the liver or circulate in the bloodstream until they are taken up by cells that need fuel. Vitamins, minerals, and other *micronutrients* (nutrients that take part in bodily processes but are not burned for energy) are absorbed and circulated in a similar way.

Important parts of the metabolic process then happen in microscopic power plants called *mitochondria* that exist in almost every cell in your body. About 2,500 mitochondria sit within each kind of cell in the body (except for red blood cells), and some cells can increase the numbers of mitochondria they have if the body perceives a need for more energy. For example, muscle cells create more mitochondria over time if you increase the energy demands on the muscles with an aerobic exercise program.

Energy is produced in the mitochondria by the breaking apart of the bonds that hold fuel molecules together. That energy is stored in the form of a molecule called *adenosine triphosphate,* or ATP, and is released as needed by the splitting apart of the ATP molecule into adenosine diphospate (ADP) and inorganic phosphorus. Think of ATP as the workhorse of the cell, supplying the energy for whatever cellular work needs to be done. For a muscle cell, this could be contraction; for an immune cell, it could be killing off bacterial invaders; for one of the cells that make up the intestinal lining, it could be bringing nutrients into and out of the bloodstream.

This conversion of food to energy is driven by a series of chemical reactions set in motion by *enzymes*—complex molecules that regulate the rate of chemical reactions in the body. Micronutrients such as vitamins and minerals act as *coenzymes* and *cofactors* in the mitochondria, working alongside the enzymes to keep energy production going.

Figure 3.1 is a diagram that represents the metabolic processes that take place in the mitochondria. It may look complicated at first, but as you read on, you will find that it is simpler than it looks.

Every fuel that goes into your body—protein, fat, or carbohydrate—is eventually transformed into a single substance, called *acetyl coenzyme A (acetyl co-A)* (5), before it is metabolized in the mitochondria. This allows

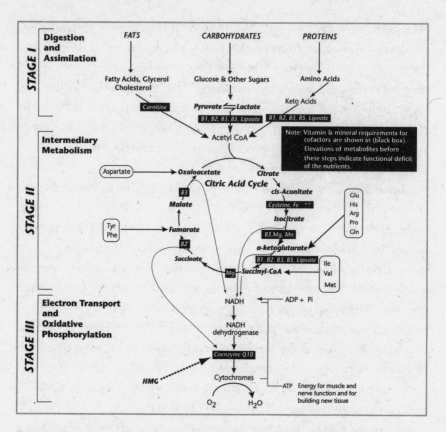

Figure 3.1 SUMMARY OF HOW FOOD IS TRANSFORMED INTO CELLULAR ENERGY
The diagram above summarizes how the three major nutrients—proteins, carbohydrates, and fats—are metabolized to provide cellular energy.

these three different types of fuel to enter the same mitochondrial energy-making process. To become acetyl co-A, glucose (blood sugar) undergoes a process termed *glycolysis* (2), fats undergo *beta-oxidation* (3), and proteins undergo *deamination* (1). The resulting acetyl co-A is a fuel that is transformed into ATP through the processes of the *citric acid cycle* and the *electron transport chain.* Once all of this has taken place, metabolic waste, in the form of carbon dioxide and water, is all that is left of the fuel that started out as (hopefully) a nutritious meal.

In glycolysis, molecules of glucose are transformed into a substance called *pyruvic acid,* or *pyruvate.* This process does not require oxygen, and so is called *anaerobic* (without oxygen) metabolism. This transformation, which requires the presence of vitamins B_1 (thiamin) and B_3 (niacin), yields two units of ATP (physiological energy) and leaves behind two molecules of pyruvate for each available molecule of glucose. Glycolysis produces energy quickly but inefficiently. Anaerobic metabolism is like trying to keep a fire going with nothing but tiny twigs. The flames shoot up quickly, but go out quickly. Glycolysis—anaerobic energy production—is often involved in the fight-or-flight reaction, a response to stress that mobilizes the body for a very fast expenditure of energy. The classic fight-or-flight example is that of a person who encounters a predator, such as a lion, in the wild—and who must then immediately either run from or fight the danger. Anaerobic metabolism helps to provide the quick energy release that helps us to respond to emergency situations. After the emergency is over, the body should be able to return to aerobic metabolism for the majority of its energy.

Approximately 90 percent of the body's energy production should be aerobic, taking place within the mitochondria. Assuming the conditions are right, the end result of glycolysis—pyruvate—is first converted into acetyl co-A. (If the cells do not have enough oxygen available, however, they may convert pyruvate into another substance, lactic acid [lactate], which is usually involved in anaerobic energy production.) Acetyl co-A enters into the series of biochemical reactions known as the citric acid cycle, or Krebs cycle, and the electron transport chain (ETC). Here it is acted on by several enzymes and nutrient coenzymes to generate energy in the form of ATP. By the time the cycle has run its course, all that is left of the original molecule of glucose is carbon dioxide, water, and thirty-six units of ATP. This portion of the energy production process is aerobic—in other words, it requires oxygen—and it is obviously much more efficient than glycolysis, since it yields thirty-six ATP units for each original glucose molecule, while glycolysis yields only two. In addition to oxygen, the citric acid cycle requires the presence of adequate amounts of of certain nutrients, among them vitamins B_1 (thiamin), B_2 (riboflavin), and B_3 (niacin); lipoic acid; pantothenic acid; the minerals iron, magnesium, manganese, phosphorus, and sulfur; and the amino acids arginine, aspartic acid, cysteine, glutamic acid, glutamine, histidine, isoleucine, methionine, phenylalanine, proline, tyrosine, and valine. The electron transport chain, which is the other energy (ATP)–producing metabolic pathway within the mitochondria, helps to produce another three units of ATP. This process requires the presence of coenzyme Q_{10}, magnesium, zinc, and vitamins B_2, B_3, C, and K.

Another nutrient, called carnitine, serves as a sort of shuttle for fatty acid molecules, transporting them across the membranes that surround the mitochondria so that they can be transformed into acetyl co-A and used for aerobic metabolism. Carnitine is made in the body from the amino acids lysine and methionine, with the help of iron and vitamins B_3, B_6, and C.

Now you can understand why nutritional deficiencies can affect one's energy and sense of well-being at the most basic level.

Aerobic energy production is the slow-burning counterpart to anaerobic energy production—the big logs on the fire that take a little longer to catch but that last for hours. You need the twigs to get those logs going, however, just as you need glycolysis (or deamination, or beta-oxidation) to make aerobic energy in the mitochondria.

The conditions are right for aerobic metabolism when *all* of the nutrients needed for the citric acid cycle and electron transport chain are readily available. If they aren't, the cell can still make energy through glycolysis— the first step shown in Figure 3.1. The problem is that this only creates two units of ATP from each original glucose molecule rather than the thirty-six made via the citric acid cycle and the three from the ETC. This is important because mitochondrial energy production shifts into this less efficient mode when the nutrient cofactors necessary for aerobic metabolism are not present in adequate amounts. Another way to look at this is that if the body lacks the necessary nutrients to fuel these metabolic pathways, fewer mitochondria are able to produce the high amounts of ATP that the citric acid cycle and electron transport chain yield.

THE FAR-REACHING EFFECTS
OF INEFFICIENT ENERGY PRODUCTION

When the mitochondria produce energy inefficiently, the adrenal glands and thyroid gland pump out more of their hormones in an effort to get more fuel to the cells. While this will give you energy, it is not the kind of energy that feels good; it is a "fight-or-flight" kind of energy that feels stressful and further depletes your body. (A more detailed discussion of adrenal and thyroid hormones appears in Chapter 9.) Your muscles, which are your body's main storage depot for glucose, become depleted as the adrenal and thyroid hormones cause them to give up their stored fuel to be burned by cells throughout the body.

The brain has an especially high requirement for glucose; along with the red blood cells (which carry oxygen through the bloodstream), it uses up about 65 percent of the glucose circulating in the blood. If your body is burning glucose inefficiently, your brain may not get as much glucose as it needs, possibly leading to the "brain fog" that is so common in new moms, and that is often chalked up to sleep deprivation.

If pyruvate, the end product of glycolysis, is not transformed into acetyl co-A and handed on down to the processes of aerobic metabolism, it is transformed into lactic acid. This can happen due either to anaerobic exercise—exercise that raises the heart rate too high—which causes the body to burn glucose, or to a deficiency of the B vitamins required to convert the pyruvate into acetyl co-A and move it through the citric acid cycle and electron transport chain. The presence of excessive levels of lactic acid in the body can have a number of different effects. Lactic acid buildup stimulates the adrenal glands to produce the stress hormone cortisol, leading to even more losses of glucose from the muscles, more glycolysis, and less aerobic energy production in the cells. Excessive cortisol production in turn also induces the body to break down tissues and reduce the production of other important hormones and of the neurotransmitter serotonin—all of which can have negative effects throughout the body as well as on mood. Lactic acid buildup also causes a distinctive fatigued sensation in the muscles—you may have felt the "burn" of lactic acid buildup in your muscles during heavy exercise. A subtler, chronic form of lactic acid buildup can occur if the nutrients your mitochondria need for aerobic metabolism are scarce. If you tend to awaken in the middle of the night and have trouble going back to sleep, lactic acid buildup could be the cause. Fatigue, the shakes and sweats of low blood sugar (hypoglycemia), and cravings for sweets all can be signs that your cells are using up your body's glucose stores too quickly. Many people with chronic fatigue syndrome, fibromyalgia, and physiologic depression have problems with lactic acid buildup.

Medical research has linked chronic fatigue syndrome, fibromyalgia (a mysterious chronic muscle pain syndrome), migraine headaches, heart rate irregularities, and diabetes to mitochondrial dysfunction. Our own clinical experience has shown that supplying plenty of the right nutrients can do wonders for postpartum fatigue by supplying the mitochondria with the fuel they need to burn energy efficiently. (In later chapters, you will find guidelines for increasing your intake of these nutrients with diet and supplements.)

CONTROLLING FREE-RADICAL PRODUCTION

Just as your car makes toxic exhaust during the process of fuel combustion, the mitochondria make their own potentially toxic byproducts in the process of metabolism. These byproducts are *free radicals,* and they can do significant damage in the body if produced in excess, or if the body is unable to remove them safely. Free-radical production is escalated under certain circumstances, such as when your immune system goes on the attack (either against harmful organisms or, in the case of autoimmune disease, against the body's own tissues), when your liver filters out and disposes of toxic substances, or when you are under a great deal of physical or emotional stress. Free-radical overload is thought to play a role in causing many, if not most, chronic and serious diseases, including cancer, heart disease, and Alzheimer's disease, as well as in the aging process.

Your body employs substances known as *antioxidants* to protect itself against free radicals. Vitamins C and E and beta-carotene are well-known antioxidants found in the foods you eat. Dozens of other antioxidants are found in healthy foods as well. Study after study has shown that people who eat diets rich in antioxidants are healthier than those who do not. A shortage of these nutrients allows excess free radicals to age you prematurely, inside and out. (Dietary measures to increase your supply of antioxidant nutrients will be discussed in Chapter 5.)

Your body also makes its own antioxidants, including the enzymes glutathione, superoxide dismutase, catalase, and coenzyme Q_{10}. However, it can produce these substances only with the aid of certain nutrients from foods, including the amino acid cysteine and the minerals selenium, manganese, copper, zinc, and iron. If the supply of any of these nutrient *precursors* (building blocks) is insufficient, antioxidant production suffers and free radicals can begin to build up and cause damage.

System 2: Detoxification

The detoxification systems are your body's cleanup crew. Whenever a potentially harmful substance needs to be removed from the body, these systems are called upon to do the job.

Toxins originate both within and outside of the body. Some toxins are created in the natural course of metabolism; hormones and other biochemicals made by the body do not float around in your system indefinitely, but are broken down and eliminated once they have served their purpose. Chemicals with which you come in contact daily—such as cleaning solutions, medicines, car exhaust, and preservatives in foods, among many others—are also processed and eliminated by your body's detoxification systems. Even nutrients from healthy foods must be processed in the liver, a key part of the detoxification system, before they exit the body.

In an ideal world—with plenty of organic sugar- and additive-free food, a relaxed lifestyle, no need for medicines, and no pollution—your body's detoxification systems would have a reasonable workload. Unfortunately, we do not live in such a world, and we're guessing that you don't either.

Processed foods such as breads, cakes, cookies, chips, luncheon meats, condiments, and sauces tend to be loaded with preservatives, flavorings, stabilizers, and other substances that must be broken down by your body and discharged. Every time you take a medication or are exposed to a chemical, it has to be processed and eliminated from your system. This is why it is important to keep your detoxification systems running smoothly. If they cannot do their job adequately, toxins can build up in your body,

effectively gumming up the works at the cellular level. Having poorly op-
erating detoxification systems can lead to fatigue and decreased immunity
by affecting the functioning of mitochondria and increasing free-radical
production. Over the long term, they may increase your risk of developing cancer, neurological diseases such as Alzheimer's disease or Parkinson's disease, and other chronic disorders. For example, recent studies
have shown a direct link between exposure to pesticides over the years and
Parkinson's disease.

THE LIVER: YOUR BEST ALLY AGAINST TOXINS

Most detoxification processes happen in the liver, intestines, and kidneys.
Like all of the systems we talk about in this chapter, the detoxifying organs require specific nutrients to do their jobs. The most active detoxica-
tion organ, the liver, is the largest solid organ in the body. If it is given the
right raw materials, it does an amazing job of filtering toxins out of the
blood, altering them to make them less toxic, and, eventually, sending
them out of the body as waste.

Traditional Chinese medicine (TCM) and other traditional schools of
medicine teach the importance of a healthy liver for overall wellness, but
conventional medicine has yet to appreciate the ways in which detoxification can set the stage for true healing. In fact, conventional medicine usually treats illness by prescribing drugs, which *increase* the stress on the
liver. This is one of the reasons why most drug therapies for chronic postpartum illnesses fall short of effecting a cure.

The subtle but important differences between one person's body and
another's—in other words, biochemical individuality—really show up
when it comes to liver function. While one person's liver might be able to
meet the detoxification demands of a highly polluted environment and
a junk-food diet, another person's may be overwhelmed by ordinary
everyday exposure to seemingly normal chemicals such as cleaning products. While one person may take a given medication and do just fine, another person may suffer intense side effects from the same drug. These
differences can be traced back to the detoxification ability of each person's
liver. Whether you find yourself at one end or the other of the detox spec-

trum, or somewhere in the middle, you can improve your liver's ability to detoxify by ensuring that it has all of the nutrients it needs to do its job.

Blood that has just absorbed nutrients from the intestines is channeled directly to the liver to be filtered for toxins. In the time it took you to read the last two paragraphs, roughly two quarts of blood passed through your liver. If your liver is functioning well, any drugs, foreign chemicals such as pesticides, "used-up" hormones and other biochemicals, and toxins made within the digestive tract were filtered out of that blood. Before many of these toxins can be flushed out of your body, they must undergo two distinct detoxification phases in the liver, designated phase I and phase II. Both phases have to be in good working order for detoxification to proceed smoothly, and in order for this to happen, key nutrients are needed in adequate amounts. Genetics and the lifetime toxic workload placed on your liver also affect how well your liver runs through each phase.

The following section describes the two phases of detoxification in some technical detail. The purpose of this is not to have you memorize a lot of new biochemistry, but rather to demonstrate how essential nutrients are to each step in the process of eliminating toxins from your body. If your body is not eliminating toxins effectively you are at higher risk for health problems of all kinds.

PHASE I DETOXIFICATION

In this phase, a group of 50 to 100 specialized enzymes alter toxins to prepare them for phase II. The molecular structure of the toxin is changed in a way that readies it to be changed further during the next step of the detoxification process. We like to think of phase I as the *activation* step. Phase I has three basic ways to neutralize toxic chemicals:

1. It can change the chemical structure of a toxic molecule so that it can be dissolved in water.
2. It can break a toxic chemical into two or more less toxic or harmless chemicals.
3. It can change a toxic molecule into a different type of molecule so that other enzymes can detoxify it more easily.

Activated toxins—toxins that have been through phase I liver detoxification—are sometimes more toxic than the original compound, so it is very important that they be moved into phase II. In some instances, a substance that does not cause cancer *becomes* carcinogenic after activation, and is then neutralized in phase II. This is true of some hormones that must undergo detoxification to be eliminated from the body. Thus, if phase I is accelerated or phase II is slowed down, activated toxins build up and can damage the liver or pass out of the liver into the general circulation. If phase I is slowed down, the liver becomes unable to keep up with detoxification demands. You can think of this as a stream that cascades over two waterfalls, with a cold, clear pond between them. When the water flows steadily, the pond remains clear and clean. If the second waterfall is clogged, the pond becomes stagnant until it overflows, carrying debris into the stream below it. If the first waterfall becomes clogged, the flow backs up and stagnates above it as the pond below dries up.

Alcohol, tobacco smoke, and some medications (for example, the steroid drug prednisone) have the effect of speeding up phase I detoxification. So do the toxins found in charcoal-broiled meats. Many environmental toxins, including chemicals in car exhaust, paint, nail polish, and pesticides, also rev up phase I, potentially causing an accumulation of activated toxins in the body.

The key here is to maintain *balance* between the two parts of the detoxification system. The best ways to do that are to avoid toxic substances whenever possible and to supply your body with all of the nutrients it needs to run smoothly through both phases. As long as phase II can keep up with phase I, some acceleration may be more helpful than harmful. Some highly nutritious foods speed up phase I. The cruciferous vegetables—broccoli, Brussels sprouts, cabbage, cauliflower, and their relatives—have this effect.

The most popular drug treatments for postpartum depression, including fluoxetine (Prozac) and other drugs in its class, slow down phase I detoxification. So do the benzodiazepine tranquilizers, such as alprazolam (Xanax), diazepam (Valium), and lorazepam (Ativan); many antibiotics; antihistamines given for allergies; and stomach-acid blockers such as cimetidine (Tagamet) and ranitidine (Zantac). When drugs inhibit phase I detoxification, other toxins (including other drugs) can build up to harmful levels because of the liver's decreased ability to get rid of them.

Phase I can also be inhibited by nutritious foods. Grapefruit juice contains a substance that inhibits phase I enzymes so strongly that it can cause drug overdoses. The enzymes are slowed so much that they cannot detoxify drugs fast enough, and the levels of the drug in the bloodstream climb too high. Capsaicin, the compound that makes hot peppers hot, also slows down phase I. The common spice turmeric, found most commonly in curry powder, slows down phase I while egging on phase II, an effect that can help to move toxins more quickly through the two phases. This may explain turmeric's powerful anticancer properties.

Certain nutrients act as coenzymes to the phase I detoxifying enzymes. Vitamins B_2, B_3, B_6, and B_{12}, plus folic acid, bioflavonoids, branched-chain amino acids, and phospholipids are needed to keep phase I going smoothly. If some of these nutrients sound unfamiliar to you, don't worry. You will learn everything you need to know about them later on. Our goal here is to show you how nutrients keep your body systems working smoothly. We will get to specifics about those nutrients—and ways to tell whether you need more of them—later in the book.

The more detoxifying work phase I has to do, the more free radicals it produces. Liver tissues can end up being damaged by these free radicals if there aren't enough antioxidants available to handle them. Vitamin C, beta-carotene, vitamin E, coenzyme Q_{10}, and the minerals copper, manganese, selenium, and zinc are all needed to prevent free-radical overload in the liver. Substances known as *thiol compounds,* which are found in garlic, onions, and the cruciferous vegetables, add to the liver's antioxidant power. Bioflavonoids and anthocyanidins are other nutrients that help to quench free radical fires.

PHASE II DETOXIFICATION

During phase II detoxification, activated substances from phase I—otherwise known as *intermediates*—are altered further. Seven different major biochemical reactions occur in this phase, known as glutathione conjugation, amino acid conjugation, methylation, sulfation, acetylation, glu-curonidation, and sulfoxidation. Each of these reactions works on specific types of intermediates and needs specific nutrients in order to proceed to successful completion. Basically, these reactions work by adding a mole-cule to the intermediate from phase I, making it less toxic and soluble in water. Then the final product can be flushed out of the body in either the urine or the bile, another product of the liver. Bile leaves the body as part of solid waste.

The nutrients required for phase II fall into two categories. The first are the amino acids, which donate molecules that are attached to phase I intermediates. These include the sulfur donors, among which are the amino acids methionine, taurine, cysteine, and N-acetylcysteine. Other, non-sulfur-containing amino acids are also required: glycine, glutamine, ornithine, and arginine. The antioxidant amino acid glutathione is also required for phase II detoxification.

The following is a brief summary of the individual phase II processes, the types of toxins they are used to eliminate, and the nutrients required for them to be carried out properly:

- *Acetylation* is a phase II liver detoxification pathway that attaches acetyl co-A to toxins to make them far less harmful and easy to excrete. This process requires vitamin B_2, pantothenic acid, molybdenum, and vitamin C to function properly.
- *Amino acid conjugation* helps the body to rid itself of many toxic chemicals, called *xenobiotics,* from the environment. The amino acids glycine, taurine, glutamine, arginine, and ornithine must be available for this liver detoxification pathway to function properly. Amino acids are available in protein-rich foods if they are eaten in adequate amounts.
- *Glucuronidation* helps to detoxify many prescription drugs and, to some extent, the reproductive and adrenal hormones. Glu-curonidation requires magnesium and vitamin B_6.
- *Glutathione conjugation* helps to detoxify and eliminate poisons in the liver, lungs, intestines, and kidneys. Glutathione is one of the most important antioxidants and anticarcinogens in the

body. Its synthesis requires adequate amounts of the amino acids cysteine, glutamic acid, and glycine. Nutrients that help to raise glutathione levels include vitamin C, alpha-lipoic acid, N-acetylcysteine whey protein, and the amino acids glutamine and methionine.

- *Methylation* helps to detoxify many of the steroid hormones, including estrogen. The methylation pathway begins with the amino acid methionine, and needs vitamin B_{12}, folic acid, choline, and vitamin B_6 to function properly. Methylation eventually yields usable sulfate with the help of the trace mineral molybdenum.

- *Sulfation* is the main liver detoxification pathway that neutralizes the stress hormone cortisol, as well as many environmental toxins, food additives, microbial products, and some commonly prescribed drugs. Usable sulfur is needed for sulfation to run unimpeded. Sources of sulfur include the sulfur-bearing amino acids methionine and cysteine, and the nutritional product methylsulfonylmethane (MSM).

- *Sulfoxidation* transforms toxic sulfite molecules into sulfate with the assistance of the mineral molybdenum. This is the last part of the methylation process (see above). Sulfites are compounds that are added to some foods to preserve freshness. For example, they are often found in wine, dried fruit, dehydrated foods, seasonings, and salad dressings. Many restaurants use them on salad bar foods. Ironically, sulfites, which can be highly allergenic and can interfere with breathing in those who are sensitive to them, are also added to some asthma medications.

A diet low in protein—all too common in women who are trying to lose weight with a low-fat diet—can dramatically slow phase II detoxification. Aspirin and other nonsteroidal anti-inflammatory drugs (NSAIDs), including ibuprofen (found in Advil, Nuprin, and other products), also slow phase II detoxification.

Does even the smallest bit of caffeine keep you wide awake at night? You could have sluggish phase I detox. Can you guzzle two cups of coffee

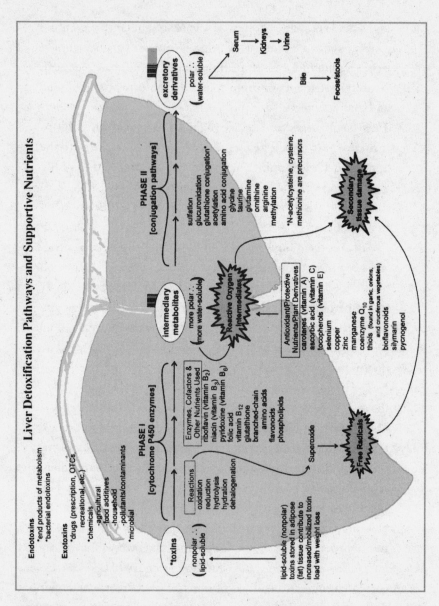

Figure 3.2 LIVER DETOXIFICATION PATHWAYS AND SUPPORTIVE NUTRIENTS
The diagram above summarizes the major liver detoxification pathways and the nutrients required for them to be completed successfully.

in the afternoon and sleep just fine? Your phase I enzymes might be over-active. Does garlic make you sick? Does your urine have a strong smell after you eat asparagus? Did you suffer from toxemia during your pregnancy? Any of these symptoms may indicate problems with phase II. Specially targeted nutrients can do wonders for your liver's detoxifying ability. (See Figure 3.2 for an illustration of the liver detoxification pathways and the nutrients needed for them to operate properly.) We will explain how to support liver detoxification with diet and supplements in Chapters 5 and 7.

Fat Balance

Underlying a wide range of the postpartum ailments we often see in our practices—including allergies, asthma, autoimmune diseases, eczema, and depression and other mood problems—is a single nutritional imbalance: too much of certain types of fats and not enough of others. This imbalance is rampant in the modern world because of the ways in which our diets have changed over the past century.

You may be accustomed to thinking of fat only in terms of how much of it has collected on certain parts of your body, preventing you from getting into your prepregnancy jeans. Or you may only consider it when loading up your shopping cart with low-fat or nonfat foods. If so, it is time to change your thinking.

Certain fats are essential for life. Every cell in your body is surrounded by a membrane made from fatty acids, the most basic building blocks of fats. (From this point forward, for simplicity's sake, we will use the terms *fatty acids* and *fats* interchangeably.) Fats are necessary building blocks for hormones. Messengers called *prostaglandins* that regulate important processes throughout the body—including immune-system and reproductive function, the inflammatory response, the constriction and expansion of blood vessels, and blood clotting—are made exclusively from fats.

During pregnancy, your body was literally drained of the fats needed for the building of your baby's brain and nervous system. The human brain is more than 60 percent fat. Research has shown that children who breastfeed score higher on intelligence quotient (I.Q.) tests than those fed formula, and many experts believe this is because mother's milk contains specific fats that are important for proper brain development. Thus, fats continue to flow from your body into the body and brain of your child during the months or years of breastfeeding. This is why taking special care to maintain a proper fatty acid balance in your own body is so important both during and after pregnancy. Not only do you need to supply your baby with enough of these brain-building fats, you also need to replenish your own supply to keep *your* brain and body in top working condition.

Research studies have shown that problems as varied as asthma, autoimmune diseases, depression, skin problems, and emotional ups and downs may improve when a healthy fatty acid balance is restored. Children with learning disabilities, attention deficit and hyperactivity disorders, and autism often improve when given fats that promote this balance as well.

ESSENTIAL FATS

Two important families of fats are the *omega-3* and *omega-6 essential fatty acids*. Nutrients that are designated *essential* are needed for survival and also cannot be made by the body and so must be supplied by the diet. (Keep in mind, though, that nutrients that can be made in the body may not be made in adequate amounts to maintain balance under certain conditions, and so can be *conditionally* essential.) A century ago, most people ate a diet that supplied somewhere between a 1:1 and a 4:1 ratio of omega-6 fats to omega-3 fats. Today, the omega-6 to omega-3 ratio is closer to between 20:1 and 30:1! Let's explore some basics about these two types of dietary fat.

The omega-6 fats include *linoleic acid* (LA), found in corn, safflower, sesame, and sunflower oils; *gamma-linolenic acid* (GLA), found in black currant seed, borage, and primrose oils; and *arachidonic acid* (AA), found in dairy products, eggs, meat, and fish that live in warm waters.

The omega-3 fats are found in far fewer foods. *Alpha-linolenic acid* (ALA) can be obtained from canola, flaxseed, pumpkinseed, and walnut oils; *eicosapentaenoic acid* (EPA) from algae and some cold-water fish; and *docosahexaenoic acid* (DHA) from some cold-water fish and algae.

THE TRANSFORMATION OF ESSENTIAL FATS
INTO PROSTAGLANDINS

The form in which you choose to eat your fats—as broiled salmon, margarine, flaxseeds, corn oil, french fries, or chicken-fried steak—will have dramatic effects on how you think, feel, learn, and remember. Your choice of fats also powerfully influences the formation of prostaglandins, hormonelike substances that regulate many body systems. Before we get into the details of how this works, let's examine how the food you put into your mouth is transformed into prostaglandins.

Figure 3.3 is a diagram showing different types of essential fatty acids and the prostaglandins they can be used to produce (as well as which other

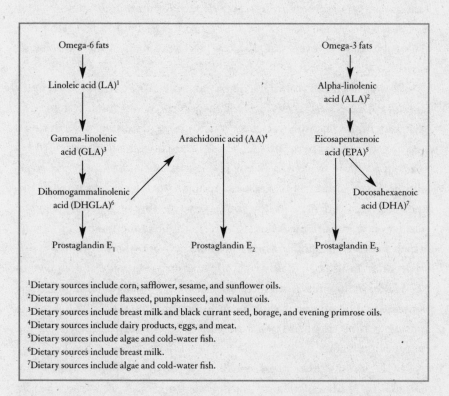

Omega-6 fats

Linoleic acid (LA)[1]

Gamma-linolenic acid (GLA)[3]

Arachidonic acid (AA)[4]

Dihomogammalinolenic acid (DHGLA)[6]

Prostaglandin E$_1$

Omega-3 fats

Alpha-linolenic acid (ALA)[2]

Eicosapentaenoic acid (EPA)[5]

Docosahexaenoic acid (DHA)[7]

Prostaglandin E$_2$

Prostaglandin E$_3$

[1]Dietary sources include corn, safflower, sesame, and sunflower oils.
[2]Dietary sources include flaxseed, pumpkinseed, and walnut oils.
[3]Dietary sources include breast milk and black currant seed, borage, and evening primrose oils.
[4]Dietary sources include dairy products, eggs, and meat.
[5]Dietary sources include algae and cold-water fish.
[6]Dietary sources include breast milk.
[7]Dietary sources include algae and cold-water fish.

Figure 3.3 RELATIONSHIPS AMONG ESSENTIAL FATTY ACIDS AND PROSTAGLANDINS
The diagram above represents the transformation of various omega-3 and omega-6 fatty acids into other fatty acids and, ultimately, into prostaglandins.

fatty acids they can be transformed into). As with essential fatty acids, there are various families of prostaglandins, designated series 1, series 2, and series 3—or, more simply, prostaglandin E_1, E_2, and E_3. Figure 3.3 represents a somewhat simplified version—there are many more prostaglandins than are listed here—but it should serve to give you a general impression of the various classes of these biochemicals and how they check and balance one another. All of these prostaglandins are necessary and perform valuable functions; none is purely "good" or "bad." The important point is that they need to be in balance with one another, and that the nutrients you take in—fats as well as other nutrients that affect the processes shown in Figure 3.3—have a direct impact on that state of balance.

That said, we will at times refer to "good" or "bad" prostaglandins. Because the typical American diet contains excessive amounts of the fats that go to form prostaglandin E_2 (PGE_2), they end up sending the body out of balance. That is why the PGE_2 precursors tend to be cast as nutritional bad guys, even though those fats play many valuable roles in the body.

Prostaglandins E_1 and E_3 (PGE_2 and PGE_3) generally have anti-inflammatory effects, meaning that they keep the immune system's response to injury or insult in check. When a foreign substance is identified by your immune system, it is tagged for destruction and neutralized by specialized immune cells. Wherever these immune cells gather in large numbers, the inflammatory process results. An infected cut that swells and reddens is inflamed. When you have a cold, the linings of your nasal passages become inflamed. Fever is a form of the inflammatory process in which your whole body is warmed to help activate your immune system. Inflammation also happens in response to injury—a swollen knot on your head after it has been bumped, or a swollen ankle after it has been sprained. Inflammation is your immune system doing the job of cleaning house—getting rid of foreign, damaged, or dead tissues to make way for new, healthy tissues.

PGE_2, on the other hand, escalates the inflammatory process. If inflammation escalates too far, tissue damage and free-radical overload can result. Thus, if there is too much PGE_2 and not enough PGE_1 and PGE_3, inflammation can run amok. Allergies, asthma, eczema, joint pain, and autoimmune diseases are all manifestations of inflammation that is not being shut off at the appropriate time. In a woman who has recently given birth and is breastfeeding, and therefore is giving up PGE_1- and PGE_3-forming fats to her baby, this kind of imbalance can easily spin out of control. In the worst-case scenario, she may not even get enough of the right fats to give her baby what she needs. This could make the baby more vulnerable to allergies, asthma, eczema, and even attention deficit/hyperactivity disorder and other learning disabilities later in life.

THE ENZYME GATEKEEPERS

The availability of the right fats is not the only nutritional factor in prostaglandin formation. Several enzymes take part in the process that transforms fats into prostaglandins. These enzymes act as gatekeepers, channeling fats into the making of this or that prostaglandin. Like all the other enzymes in the body, these enzymes require specific nutrient coenzymes to do their jobs.

Aspirin and similar drugs work to reduce inflammation by affecting these enzymes, temporarily shutting down the production of both inflammatory and anti-inflammatory prostaglandins. As you will see, diet and supplements can be used in a more specific way, enhancing the balance of "good" and "bad" prostaglandins rather than just shutting them all off.

Figure 3.4 is a diagram showing which enzymes are involved in the processes that transform specific fatty acids into certain prostaglandins. As you can see, the enzyme delta-6-desaturase acts on the omega-6 fat linoleic acid (LA, found in most vegetable, nut, and seed oils) to transform it to gamma-linolenic acid (GLA). This enzyme also transforms the omega-3 fat alpha-linolenic acid (ALA) into stearidonic acid (SDA), which then is transformed (by the enzyme elongase) into eicosapentaenoic acid (EPA). EPA is the fat that supports the production of prostaglandin E_3 (PGE_3) and the formation of brain cells. GLA is used to make anti-inflammatory prostaglandin E_1 (PGE_1) and also supports healthy nervous system function.

The activity of delta-6-desaturase is affected by dietary factors. The consumption of too much saturated fat (found in meat, dairy products, fried foods, and most junk food), too much alcohol, or too much sugar or

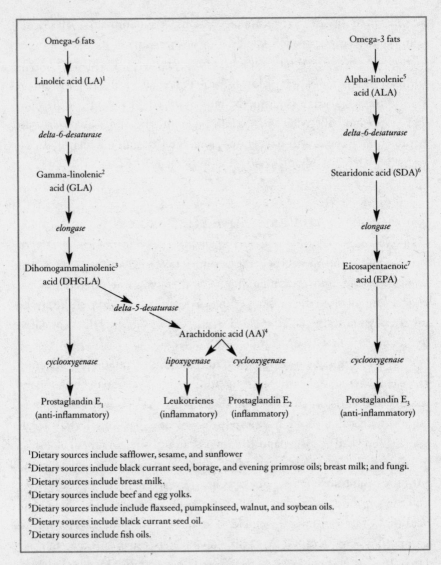

Omega-6 fats

Linoleic acid (LA)[1]

delta-6-desaturase

Gamma-linolenic[2]
acid (GLA)

elongase

Dihomogammalinolenic[3]
acid (DHGLA)

delta-5-desaturase

Arachidonic acid (AA)[4]

cyclooxygenase

Prostaglandin E$_1$
(anti-inflammatory)

lipoxygenase

Leukotrienes
(inflammatory)

cyclooxygenase

Prostaglandin E$_2$
(inflammatory)

Omega-3 fats

Alpha-linolenic[5]
acid (ALA)

delta-6-desaturase

Stearidonic acid (SDA)[6]

elongase

Eicosapentaenoic[7]
acid (EPA)

cyclooxygenase

Prostaglandin E$_3$
(anti-inflammatory)

[1]Dietary sources include safflower, sesame, and sunflower
[2]Dietary sources include black currant seed, borage, and evening primrose oils; breast milk; and fungi.
[3]Dietary sources include breast milk.
[4]Dietary sources include beef and egg yolks.
[5]Dietary sources include include flaxseed, pumpkinseed, walnut, and soybean oils.
[6]Dietary sources include black currant seed oil.
[7]Dietary sources include fish oils.

Figure 3.4 Enzymes Involved in the Formation of Prostaglandins from Omega-3 and Omega-6 Fats
The diagram above represents the process through which omega-3 and omega-6 fats are transformed into prostaglandins, indicating which enzymes are involved in each step (all of the italicized words ending in -*ase* are the names of enzymes).

refined flour all conspire to slow this enzyme down. High stress levels also inhibit its activity. Trans-fatty acids (TFAs), found in the hydrogenated oils present in most processed foods, are particularly notorious for slowing down the activity of delta-6-desaturase. Hydrogenated oils are produced by subjecting vegetable oils to a process aptly called *hydrogenation,* which involves the bombardment of liquid oils with hydrogen atoms to make them solid and prevent them from spoiling. Hydrogenation has enabled food manufacturers to greatly extend the shelf life of the vegetable oils used to make processed foods.

The trans-fatty acids created by hydrogenation disrupt the balance of the other fats. They have harmful effects on the stability of cell membranes and the structure of nerve and brain cells. They interfere with the formation of anti-inflammatory prostaglandins. Trans fats pass readily into a nursing mother's milk supply, so the more of them she eats, the more her baby eats. If you want to avoid them—and you should, as much as you possibly can—read labels before buying any processed foods. Trans-fatty acids usually show up on food labels as *partially hydrogenated vegetable oils.* They are present in almost all breads, chips, cookies, frozen entrées, pastries, salad dressings, and sauces.

Large amounts of alpha-linolenic acid (ALA) in your diet can also subdue delta-6-desaturase activity. Some experts say that adding lots of flaxseeds and flaxseed oil to your diet will enhance the production of anti-inflammatory prostaglandins, but we recommend you use flaxseed and other ALA-rich foods in moderation. By suppressing the delta-6-desaturase enzyme, ALA suppresses both "good" and "bad" prostaglandin formation—in much the same way as aspirin does. Suppressing all of the prostaglandins creates not balance, but a different kind of imbalance. Flaxseed oil also spoils easily, and eating spoiled oil can cause excessive free radicals to form in your body. (More about flaxseeds and flaxseed oil in Chapter 7.)

If you look back at Figure 3.4 on page 56, you will see that dihomogammalinolenic acid (DHGLA), which can be formed from GLA (it can also enter your baby's body directly through your milk), can go one of two directions: It can be transformed either into "good" PGE_1 or into arachidonic acid (AA). The activity of the enzyme delta-5-desaturase determines which way this process goes. Delta-5-desaturase activity in turn is governed by two hormones, insulin and glucagon. Specifically, insulin activates it and glucagon suppresses it. The body's insulin level rises if you eat lots of sugars and refined carbohydrates (for example, breads, muffins, crackers, pretzels, pies, donuts, cakes, cookies, and the like), whereas glucagon levels rise when you eat foods that contain balanced amounts of fat and protein. At the same time, eicosapentaenoic acid (EPA), the omega-3 fat found in fish, suppresses delta-5-desaturase production. The net result, in other words: Sugars and refined carbohydrates have the effect of using DHGLA to increase AA levels and the production of "bad" prostaglandin production, while a diet rich in healthy proteins, fats, and deep-water fish has the effect of funneling DHGLA toward the production of "good" prostaglandins.

Keep in mind that AA is considered a nonessential fat—that is, the human body can make it from other fats from the age of about six months forward. During the first six months, your baby gets AA from your milk. Besides vegetable oils, what do you think is the major source of dietary fat in the typical American diet? Meats, eggs, and dairy products, all of which contain lots of AA. We don't want to make AA into the bad guy here—it is an important nutrient, and the cholesterol found in meats, eggs, and dairy products is essential to your good health. However, Americans tend to eat far more AA-containing foods than they need. We want to encourage you to strive for a more balanced approach.

The activity of two of the other enzymes mentioned in Figure 3.4—cyclooxygenase and lipoxygenase—can also be influenced by diet and supplement use. Slowing down some of these enzymes can also slow the transformation of AA into inflammatory prostaglandins and leukotrienes, which are related to the prostaglandins.

The bottom line here is that the balance of omega-3 and omega-6 fats in your cells is directly attributable to your diet and the nutritional supplements you take, and this balance, along with how the other systems in your body are working, influences the balance of inflammatory and anti-inflammatory prostaglandins made in your body. If your family has a history of inflammatory disorders such as asthma, allergies, autoimmune diseases, eczema, or heart disease, you may have a genetic predisposition to make more of the inflammatory prostaglandins, and you may have to work a little harder than other people to hit your balance point.

All of the enzymes that participate in the transformation of fats to prostaglandins require nutrient coenzymes. Vitamins A, B_3, B_6, C, and E, plus the minerals magnesium and zinc, are required in order for delta-6-desaturase to make GLA from LA and EPA from ALA. The transformation of EPA into docosahexaenoic acid (DHA) requires biotin and vitamin B_6. Once again, you can see how your nutrient status can have far-reaching effects on your health.

Nervous-System Balance

The nervous system contains more of the omega-3 fat DHA than any other tissue in the body, and the cells that make up this system do not function well when there is not enough of it to go around. Getting plenty of omega-3s and gamma-linolenic acid (GLA) can also help your mood and clarity of thinking in the postpartum months, and ensure that your baby has enough of these nutritional building blocks to build a healthy nervous system.

Nerve cells form intricate networks throughout every inch of the body. The cells of the peripheral nervous system, autonomic nervous system, and the central nervous system—made up of the spinal cord and brain—form a circuit that regulates your every body function. Information passes through this complex circuitry in the form of electrical impulses. Let's say you accidentally stub your toe on a table leg. Receptors in the nerve cells of your toe are traumatized and they start an impulse up the nerve cells of your leg. That impulse continues into your spinal cord and all the way up to your brain, where it is translated as a sensation of pain—at which point your brain prompts your body to hop away from the table, make pained noises, and sit down to rub your injured toe. Each nerve cell throughout the body is linked to many others by tiny spaces called *synapses*. Every time an impulse moves from one nerve cell to the next, it has to move across the synapse. The *neurotransmitters* are nervous system chemicals that bridge these gaps.

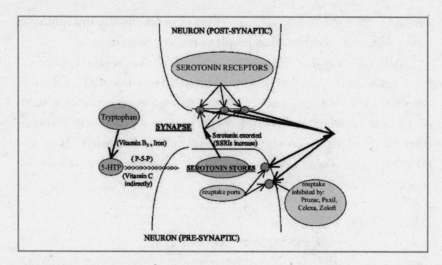

Figure 3.5 NEUROTRANSMITTER RELEASE AND UPTAKE
Impulses are transmitted from nerve cell to nerve cell by means of chemicals called neurotransmitters, which are released at the end of one nerve cell, travel across the synapse to the next nerve cell, and are then taken up by that cell. This process occurs both in nerves cells in the brain and in nerve cells in the rest of the body, resulting in the transmission of impulses to and from the brain.

When an electrical impulse moves to the end of one nerve cell, it stimulates the release of neurotransmitters into the synapse. Those neurotransmitters are then taken up by receptors on the nerve cell on the other side of the synapse, causing the impulse to shoot toward the next synapse along that particular nerve pathway. (See Figure 3.5.) Many different neurotransmitters exist, and each one has its own role in maintaining nervous system balance.

Despite the now-common belief that depression is caused by a deficiency of the neurotransmitter serotonin—which can be manipulated by fluoxetine (Prozac) and similar drugs—other neurotransmitters also have significant impact on mood and emotions. Trying to fix mood by altering a single neurotransmitter is like trying to fix a completely mismatched outfit by changing your shoes. While those new shoes might be great-looking enough to distract from the rest of your outfit, you are going to have to change more than that to create a coordinated look.

If you are a nursing mother suffering from depression, anxiety, or irritability, you want to find ways to regulate neurotransmitter levels without drugs. The good news is most mothers can accomplish this quite effectively and reliably with food, supplements, and exercise.

At this very moment, at least fifty different types of neurotransmitters are zapping through your synapses. Each and every one of these neurotransmitters are made of amino acids, the building blocks of protein, with processes that involve enzymes and nutrient cofactors. Some neurotransmitters are composed of nothing but a single amino acid, while others are made of groups of amino acids bound together. Let us turn to a discussion of a few of the major neurotransmitters.

SEROTONIN

Serotonin is probably the best-known neurotransmitter today. It is made from the amino acid tryptophan, which is found in small amounts in protein-rich foods, and pyridoxyl-5-phosphatase, the active form of vitamin B_6. Serotonin helps to regulate mood, appetite, digestive-system function, and how we experience pain. Increasing serotonin levels in the synapses of the brain can bring on feelings of well-being and suppress appetite; reducing serotonin can have the opposite effect. Serotonin is the precursor to another neurotransmitter called *melatonin,* which is your brain's very own natural sleep-inducer. Vitamin B_6, vitamin B_3, and iron are needed to transform tryptophan into serotonin, and vitamin B_{12}, folic acid, vitamin B_6, pantothenic acid, and compounds such as choline or betaine, which are known as *methyl donors,* are needed to transform serotonin into melatonin.

CATECHOLAMINES

The catecholamines are a group of three neurotransmitters—epinephrine, norepinephrine, and dopamine—that maintain your body's state of wakefulness. When you feel that "fight-or-flight" energy burst in a scary situation, catecholamines are responsible. Blood pressure, muscle movement, sex drive, immune function, learning, memory, mood, the release of various hormones, and heart, liver, lung, and intestinal function are orchestrated, in part, by the catecholamines.

All three of the catecholamines are built from the amino acids phenylalanine and tyrosine; both epinephrine and norepinephrine can be produced from dopamine. The nutrients betaine, copper, magnesium, and vitamins B_3, B_6, B_{12}, and C are used to make dopamine. A type of compound known as a *methyl donor* is also required. Wheat germ, oats, soft cheeses such as ricotta, and poultry are rich in tyrosine. Pork and wild game contain high levels of phenylalanine.

GAMMA-AMINOBUTYRIC ACID

Gamma-aminobutyric acid (GABA) is a neurotransmitter that has calming effects on the brain and body. When you take a tranquilizer such as diazepam (Valium), it relaxes you by activating GABA receptors in your brain. GABA also acts as the precursor to the sleep-inducing brain chemical gamma-hydroxybutyrate (GHB). Glutamine and glutamic acid are compounds that are very similar in structure to GABA but have opposite functions, stimulating the nervous system, thinking ability, and memory. The balance of these three neurotransmitters helps to prevent overexcitation or underexcitation of the nervous system. Glutamine, GABA, and glutamate are all made from glutamic acid. Oats, soft cheeses, ham, poultry, and wild game are all rich in glutamic acid. The enzymes that transform glutamic acid into glutamine need the mineral magnesium to do their work. The conversion of glutamic acid into GABA requires the presence of vitamin B_6.

ACETYLCHOLINE

Acetylcholine does the work of transmitting information between the nerves and muscles, controlling the tension of muscles throughout the body. It is important for thinking, mental focus, and memory. Acetylcholine levels have been found to be low in some people with age-related memory loss. Choline, a nutrient found in egg yolks, wheat germ, soy, peanuts, leafy greens, and cruciferous vegetables (see page 46), is the body's raw material for building acetylcholine. The minerals zinc and calcium and vitamins B_1, B_6, C, and pantothenic acid act as coenzymes in this process.

THE IMPORTANCE OF BALANCE

The neurotransmitters above are the stuff from which your thoughts, emotions, memories, and bodily functions are made. As with the different types of fats, all of them have important roles to play, but they must be in balance with one another. Under the best of circumstances, most people's bodies are quite adept at maintaining the right balance of these biochemicals. However, some people have a genetic predisposition that skews this balance one way or another. Disease and chronic stress also can interrupt the smooth interaction of the neurotransmitters. Some prescription drugs may rob your body of some of the nutrient precursors necessary to manufacture neurotransmitters. The first step toward neurotransmitter balance is to supply your body with the necessary amino acids, vitamins, and minerals.

In our practices, we often see mothers who are vegetarian or vegan (who eat no animal-derived foods whatsoever), and they frequently have symptoms of neurotransmitter imbalance. Some vegetarians are a bit less health-conscious than they could be, eating mostly processed foods loaded with white flour, hydrogenated fats, and sugars, and not taking care to include high-quality sources of protein in their diets. Those symptoms often disappear once they supplement their diets with amino acids—a sign that these mothers lacked the protein building blocks so essential for the building of neurotransmitters.

Nutrient depletion can disrupt the delicately balanced systems that drive your body's physical and mental processes in many different ways. When adequate nutrients are not available, the functioning of the microscopic machinery that makes you tick is compromised—setting in motion a chain of events that leads to health problems if left unchecked. In the four chapters that follow, you will find out what you can do about this. In Chapter 4, you will learn how functional deficiencies can be identified using laboratory tests, and how to interpret the results of those tests. Chapters 5 and 6 will tell you how to rebuild your nutrient reserves with diet, and Chapter 7 will enable you to do the same with nutritional supplements.

4

Laboratory Tests—
And How to Read Them

Since nutritional research started with the discovery of vitamins and minerals well over 100 years ago, it has come to be an accepted fact that all of the tissues that make up the physical body are composed of the vitamins, minerals, fats, proteins, carbohydrates, and fluids that enter your body day in and day out. In other words, you are what you eat. It naturally follows that deficiencies of key nutritional components in your tissues and the overconsumption of harmful foods that deplete nutrients are responsible for many kinds of disease processes. Treating these imbalances through dietary changes and specific supplementation of nutrients can have a profoundly beneficial effect on your health.

To zoom in more precisely on those deficiencies and imbalances, we use laboratory tests. Lab tests can measure levels of important biochemicals, nutrients, and hormones, and can help to determine the efficiency of metabolic pathways. This makes it possible to identify precise nutritional deficiencies that can then be targeted with dietary changes and with supplementation of key nutrients and hormones.

In the functional medicine, chiropractic, and traditional Chinese medicine (TCM) approaches, it is essential to see the big picture—incorporating both the patient's state of mind and the state of her body—before getting down to specific problems and solutions. The first thing to do with a new patient is to sit down for an in-depth conversation. The practitioner should become well acquainted with her health history and present state of health. A physical examination helps to further zero in on her problems. Generally, by the end of the first appointment, it should be possible to arrive at some general recommendations about supplements and changes in diet and lifestyle. For the majority of postpartum women, simply following certain basic diet and supplement recommendations should be enough to bring them back to balance and health. However, for some women, things are more complicated, and then laboratory tests can help. The results make it possible to further refine an appropriate treatment program.

This chapter should familiarize you with the general concept of laboratory testing as it is used in functional medicine. We will talk about some of the tests that are most useful for evaluation of biochemical imbalances. (Some other tests that are relevant to material in other chapters will be covered in those chapters.)

Clinical Nutrition: Linking Traditional Medicine with Modern Science

The practice of clinical nutrition—that is, the science of nutrition as applied by health-care practitioners—is far more scientifically based and advanced than most conventional doctors realize. A doctor who tells you that there is no scientific basis for nutritional medicine is literally decades behind the times. There has been and continues to be a great deal of scientific research supporting the need for specific nutritional supplementation for various health conditions. Over the past several decades, the sciences of biochemistry and research-based clinical nutrition have begun to come together to form a scientific approach to clinical nutrition. Laboratory testing to detect nutrient and hormone deficiencies has become a wonderful tool for helping patients reach optimal health.

Some of these tests are relatively new, and you may need to make an effort to seek out a doctor familiar with their use and interpretation. Others tests mentioned have been around for many years, but require the trained eye of a clinical nutrition specialist to glean the health information they can reveal. If you are fairly well informed about these tests yourself, you will be better able to find a doctor who is willing and able to use them to create the optimal nutritional prescription for your specific body. You will also be able to recommend this book to your doctor if he or she would like to know more about the tests you are asking for.

The Art of Lab Test Interpretation

Conventional physicians make extensive use of laboratory testing, but there is a twofold difference between the functional and conventional medical approaches to using lab tests. First, while both ways of practicing medicine use some of the same tests, most conventional physicians have never heard of many of the lab tests used routinely by functional medicine practitioners. Second, these two types of practitioners are likely to differ dramatically when it comes to the *interpretation* of these test results. The average conventional physician also is not likely to deeply consider the relationship between a patient's signs and symptoms—for example, depression or allergies—and subtle indicators of nutritional deficiency or hormone imbalance as seen in lab tests.

The science of laboratory testing becomes an art when it comes time to interpret the results. Every person's nutrient needs are different. Some might require higher levels of a certain nutrient than others, and what may be a very minor, nonproblematic deficiency in one person can cause significant symptoms in another. We look for *patterns* in symptoms and lab test results to discern the root problems of our patients. To some extent, you can do this yourself, and we hope to give you useful tools for doing so in this chapter and those to come. If you have read most everything up to this point, you are already on your way to identifying your specific problems. While lab tests may not be necessary for everyone, they are always useful, and can only help to pinpoint the exact deficiencies that are compromising your health.

While the conventional medical model tends to define health as the absence of disease, functional medicine and traditional Chinese medicine's vision of health is much more about sustaining *optimal* function. (A truly traditional Chinese medicine doctor gets paid only when his patients are *healthy*.) Functional medicine sees the relationship between health and disease as a continuum, not as an either/or proposition. (See Figure 4.1.)

At any point along this continuum, disease can be reversed. Wouldn't you rather catch it near the top of the continuum, before significant damage is done, than near the bottom, when extreme measures become necessary? The artful use of laboratory tests allows us to detect deficiencies and imbalances while the health problems they cause are still subtle—in other words, near the top of the continuum shown in Figure 4.1. Such imbalances and deficiencies are termed *subclinical,* which means that they are not yet causing outright disease, but will do so if not addressed. If such subclinical issues are resolved, you can reach and maintain a state of optimal health.

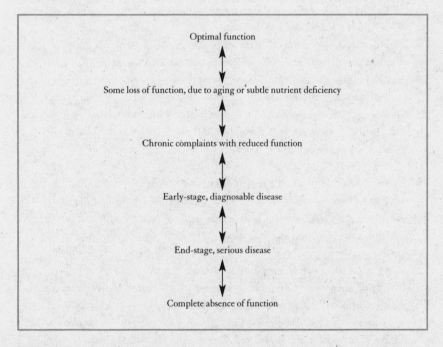

Figure 4.1 THE HEALTH-TO-DISEASE CONTINUUM
Health and disease are not true opposites, but rather exist along a continuum ranging from a complete absence of function at the lower end to optimal function at the upper end.

Karen's Story

Karen's asthma almost disappeared during her last trimester of pregnancy. It felt so good to be free of wheezes and chest tightness after suffering from them since her early twenties that she joked about wanting to stay pregnant forever.

After her son's birth, the asthma came back with a vengeance. She could barely walk a block without having to use her rescue inhaler. Also back in the picture were her hay fever, itchy eyes, and patches of red, bumpy, flaky, itchy skin on her eyelids and around her nose. She looked awful and felt worse than she looked.

She decided to go to a new allergist who had just opened up an office in town. Her son's pediatrician told her that this doctor was quite well known in the field of allergy and he might be able to help. She ended up spending an hour with a nurse who did a skin-prick test on her back, and got to talk to the doctor for only about five minutes afterward. He told her that, basically, she was allergic to everything: cats, dogs, birds, grasses, all kinds of pollen, molds, you name it. She left the allergist's office with prescriptions for steroid inhalers, one for her nose and one for her lungs, and a steroid cream for her patches of eczema. She asked him why she was so allergic now when she had never been as a kid or during her pregnancy. He said no one really knows about that, and all that can be done is to deal with the symptoms in the best way possible. He said that allergy shots sometimes work, and that she could start those while nursing if she felt like it. But the four-year commitment the shots would require sounded overwhelming to her at that point.

A friend recommended that Karen come to see me for a second opinion. We sat down for a half-hour and talked about her diet, her pregnancy, and her history of asthma and allergies. I recommended a series of tests. At her follow-up appointment, I told her that the test results appeared to show that she had food allergies, leaky gut syndrome, candida overgrowth, and low adrenal function. The allergist hadn't said a thing about any of these problems.

I recommended an elimination diet, which Karen didn't find easy to get going on, but once she had cut out basically everything but rice, vegetables, and meat, she started to feel much better. Her son's colic also disappeared within a couple of days after she eliminated wheat, dairy,

and citrus fruits from her diet. I prescribed natural hydrocortisone supplements, progesterone cream to be rubbed on her skin each night, and
supplements to help heal her digestive system, strengthen her adrenal
glands, and balance the good bowel bacteria with the bad ones. After
about two months, Karen felt and looked better than she had in years,
and was able to do fine with very occasional use of her rescue inhaler. She
also lost almost all of her twenty-five-pound pregnancy weight gain on
the new diet!

—D.R.

Laboratory Testing Basics

Lab tests can be used to assess the levels of specific nutrients and hormones
in the body. They can also be used to assess the function of organ systems.
Both types of assessment require the use of blood tests, urine tests, saliva
tests, stool tests, and/or hair analysis. To do a complete battery of lab tests,
you may need to submit urine, saliva, hair, and stool samples, in addition
to having blood drawn. Breath tests require complicated equipment and
can be done only in a health-care practitioner's office.

Different vitamins and minerals are concentrated in different tissues.
For example, the mineral magnesium is highly concentrated within red
blood cells. Therefore, measuring the level of magnesium in the *plasma*—
the watery part of the blood in which red blood cells float—does not yield
a very meaningful result. Fortunately, there is a specific test available that
can look at mineral levels within the red blood cells. Similarly, measuring
the level of the hormone progesterone in the bloodstream does not provide an accurate reflection of the activity of that hormone in the body, but
saliva or urine testing does. Amino acid levels can be measured with either
urine testing or blood plasma testing. Stool testing, urine testing, and
breath testing can yield valuable information about intestinal health that a
blood test cannot.

Chem Screen

The chem screen—short for *chemistry screen*—is a fairly general test, and is the one that a conventional doctor is likely to order for you if you go in for an annual checkup. Both conventional and functional medicine doctors look at the results of this test to diagnose or rule out pathology or serious disease. However, the typical medical doctor is not trained to read the results for what clinical nutritionists refer to as *optimal health values*. These values represent a narrower range than what is usually considered to be the "normal" or "reference" range.

A chem screen (also known as a chem panel) gives information about what is in your blood and about the functioning of your heart, lungs, kidneys, and liver. It also shows whether you have specific types of blood sugar imbalances. While other tests may be ordered along with the chem screen, often the chem screen and the patient's case history give enough information to enable a practitioner to prescribe effective therapeutic dietary and lifestyle changes.

What exactly the chem screen covers varies from practitioner to practitioner. It can include dozens of different tests. To the skilled eye of a clinical nutrition expert with functional medicine leanings, the results of these commonplace tests can reveal some very important information. The following are some of the more basic tests in the chem panel and what they can indicate. For the values considered to be low, high, and normal from a functional medicine perspective, refer to Table 4.1 on page 78.

BLOOD GLUCOSE

This test identifies abnormalities in blood sugar balance.

People who test at the *low fasting glucose level* end of the spectrum tend to need to eat something every few hours or they become dizzy and tired. This can be an indicator of *reactive hypoglycemia,* a condition caused by a lack of glucose (sugar in the blood) at the cellular level.

A *high fasting glucose level* indicates a strong possibility of a prediabetic condition or diabetes. If there are no other symptoms of diabetes, such as weight gain and other hormonal imbalances, a vitamin B₁ (thiamin) deficiency might be suspected. This is a less common cause of high blood sugar.

If glucose levels are abnormal, other tests may be recommended to more clearly identify the problem, including insulin, glycated hemoglobin, metabolic dysglycemia, or the five- or six-hour glucose tolerance test.

BLOOD UREA NITROGEN (BUN)

Urea is the main end product of protein metabolism. The blood urea nitrogen test shows the ratio of the production of urea to its clearance from the body.

Low BUN often indicates a protein or amino acid deficiency, especially in women who have recently given birth.

High BUN usually reflects some level of kidney disease.

ALBUMIN

Albumin is a protein that is produced in the liver. It is found in the blood circulating throughout your body. Measuring albumin levels can reveal much about the function of the liver and immune system.

Low albumin most often indicates a liver or immune system problem, but may also indicate digestive inflammation (often due to low stomach acid levels, especially if phosphorus is low; more about this in Chapter 8), free-radical stress, an overactive thyroid, protein deficiency, or low levels of vitamin B₁₂, C, or folic acid.

High albumin often indicates dehydration or low liver, thyroid, or adrenal function.

ALKALINE PHOSPHATASE (ALP)

ALP is an enzyme that requires zinc for its activity. It performs many functions in the body.

Low ALP is a good indication of zinc deficiency, underactive thyroid or adrenals, anemia, protein deficiency, or the use of prescription hormones (estrogens or estrogens plus androgens).

High ALP is associated with liver, bone, or intestinal problems, or with placenta problems in pregnant women. During periods of rapid bone growth, such as adolescence, or when a broken bone is healing, it is perfectly normal for ALP to rise quite a bit. However, if ALP is very high and you are not an adolescent or healing from a fracture, and you are doing your tests on your own via mail order, you should consult a physician for further testing. This could indicate any one of many potentially serious health problems, including rheumatoid arthritis, an overactive thyroid, hepatitis, or cancer.

BILIRUBIN

Bilirubin is the end product of the breakdown of hemoglobin, an iron-containing molecule that carries oxygen in the bloodstream, which takes place in the spleen, liver, and bone marrow. The liver converts bilirubin into a form that is easily flushed out of your body in the bile (which is eliminated through the bowels) or in the urine. Bilirubin is measured in three ways: total, indirect, and direct.

High bilirubin indicates liver dysfuntion. This condition causes jaundice, which results in the yellowing of skin and the whites of the eyes. A less significant elevation in bilirubin can indicate thymus dysfunction (the thymus is an immunity-regulating gland) or anemia.

CALCIUM

Levels of calcium relative to levels of phosphorus are a good indicator of low thyroid function in postpartum women. The normal ratio between calcium and phosphorus is 10:4, but in people with hypothyroidism the calcium side of the ratio rises.

High calcium can also indicate low adrenal or ovarian function, vitamin-D toxicity, or, rarely, a parathyroid gland tumor.

Low calcium is normal during pregnancy. Postpartum, it can mean low ovarian function or a deficiency of vitamin D, calcium, or protein.

CHLORIDE

Evaluating levels of chloride helps us to evaluate hydration (water balance), kidney function, and adrenal gland function. This mineral is needed for the production of hydrochloric acid in the stomach, which is essential for healthy digestion.

High chloride can indicate kidney dysfunction, excessive salt intake, overactive adrenal glands, bladder dysfunction, or dehydration.

Low chloride may indicate kidney or bowel dysfunction, low adrenal function, diabetes, or respiratory problems.

TOTAL CHOLESTEROL

The "normal" range for total cholesterol levels is 140 milligrams per deciliter (mg/dL) to 200 mg/dL of blood. Most conventional physicians tell their patients that the more they lower their cholesterol, the healthier they will be. I have often heard patients boast that their total cholesterol is 120 mg/dL or less. Their pride usually fades somewhat when I explain that such low cholesterol increases their risk of decreased immune function, and that their levels of anti-inflammatory omega-3 fats such as alpha-linolenic acid (ALA), docosahexaenoic acid (DHA), and eicosapentaenoic acid (EPA) are probably quite low. People with very low cholesterol also tend to have dry skin and are more likely to suffer from joint and muscle pain and irritable bowel syndrome than are those with higher cholesterol levels.

Cholesterol is an important substance for good health and is needed for the manufacture of brain and nerve cells and steroid hormones, including estrogen, progesterone, and cortisol. (These hormones will be discussed in detail in Chapter 9.) Cholesterol only becomes a problem if it becomes oxidized (reacts chemically with oxygen) and causes cellular damage, or if it becomes so high in concentration that it causes the blood to thicken, stressing the heart, liver, kidneys, and other important organs.

HIGH-DENSITY LIPOPROTEIN (HDL) CHOLESTEROL

HDL is actually a protein that transports the fatty substance known as cholesterol throughout the body to the liver. It is sometimes called "good cholesterol" because it has a beneficial antioxidant and anti-inflammatory effect. In other words, HDL cleans up excess cholesterol from the circulation and drops it off in the liver, where it can be processed and eliminated from the body. It helps to protect the body from too much inflammation in the arteries. Ideally, HDL should be in the 50 to 60 mg/dL range or higher, and that of the other major type of cholesterol, low-density lipoproteins (LDL), should be below 100 mg/dL. Another useful way of looking at cholesterol numbers is the ratio of total cholesterol to the protective HDL cholesterol. For example, if your total cholesterol is 180 and your HDL is 60, the ratio (60/180) is one part HDL to three parts total cholesterol, or a ratio of 3:1. You divide the total cholesterol by the HDL cholesterol. The ideal cholesterol-to-HDL ratio is less than 4:1.

Low HDL is more likely to be found in people with antioxidant deficiencies or diabetes and in users of cigarettes, steroid drugs, thiazide diuretics, or beta-blockers. People who do no aerobic exercise tend to have low HDL levels as well.

Although you may consider yourself to be too young to worry about heart disease, it is never too early to balance your HDL and LDL cholesterol levels. Heart disease develops over years and years, and if you nip it in the bud now, you can be around to see your kids have their own kids. Besides, out-of-balance blood cholesterol levels are not only indicative of heart disease risk, but are a clear sign from your body that you have not struck the right balance with your diet and lifestyle.

LOW-DENSITY LIPOPROTEIN (LDL) CHOLESTEROL

LDL picks up cholesterol in the liver, where it is made, and distributes it throughout the body. LDL cholesterol is considered "bad cholesterol" because it can become oxidized—altered by free radicals—in a way that makes it inflammatory. Oxidized cholesterol can do damage to body tissues and increases the buildup of plaque in arteries throughout the body, especially in the arteries that lead to the heart.

High LDL can indicate heart disease, insulin imbalances, antioxidant deficiencies, a genetic predisposition, low thyroid function, a diet high in carbohydrates and saturated fat, or alcoholism.

CARBON DIOXIDE (CO_2)

Carbon dioxide's job in your body is to neutralize acids.

Low CO_2 can indicate a deficiency of vitamin B_1 (thiamin) or an imbalance in the body's acid/alkaline balance, such as systemic acidosis. It can also indicate diabetes, kidney dysfunction, or dehydration.

High CO_2 can point to systemic alkalosis, adrenal hyperfunction, respiratory distress, or loss of hydrochloric acid due to vomiting. CO_2 can also be increased as a result of fever.

CREATININE

A substance in muscle tissue called creatine decomposes into creatinine when the muscle contracts. Creatinine is normally processed by the kidneys and flushed from the body through the urine.

Low creatinine may be caused by increased kidney activity during pregnancy, which causes creatinine levels to drop. Both low and high creatinine can indicate kidney disease.

High creatine can indicate kidney disease, congestive heart failure, diabetes, starvation, gout, urinary blockage, or excessive protein consumption.

GAMMA-GLUTAMYLTRANSFERASE (GGT) AND ASPARTATE AMINOTRANSFERASE (AST)

The levels of these two enzymes are sensitive indicators of liver function.

Low AST (also sometimes referred to as glutamic oxaloacetic transaminase, or GOT) can indicate vitamin B_6 anemia or protein deficiency.

High AST can be a result of heart disease, liver disease, free-radical pathology, and some infectious diseases.

A test for levels of another enzyme, alanine aminotransferase (ALT, also known as glutamate pyruvate transaminase, or GPT), is useful for identifying heart problems.

LACTATE DEHYDROGENASE (LDH)

This test measures levels of a group of enzymes involved in carbohydrate metabolism. They are found in the bloodstream and in all of the tissues of the body, but are especially important for proper function of the pancreas (which makes insulin and digestive enzymes) and the cellular machinery that metabolizes glucose.

High LDH in the blood occurs when there is damage or inflammation in the heart, kidneys, liver, skeletal muscle, or red blood cells. When we see high LDH, we suspect active infection, liver dysfunction, inflammatory disease, or heart disease, depending upon other test results and symptoms.

Low LDH is usually a sign of reactive hypoglycemia (low blood sugar).

MAGNESIUM

Because magnesium is highly concentrated within red blood cells, serum measurements—the type usually performed in a chem screen—are not very useful. Tests for magnesium levels in red blood cells (RBC) are valuable, although expensive. Magnesium is involved in more than 300 different cellular reactions. We have found that it is so frequently deficient that we generally recommend supplementation if serum levels are not above 2.0 mg/dL. A supplement of 400 milligrams of magnesium per day is often extremely helpful for many conditions.

PHOSPHORUS

Phosphorus is important for the metabolism of glucose and proper digestive function, as well as many other body functions. The body needs this mineral to make ATP, an integral part of cellular energy production.

If phosphorus is below 2.4 or above 2.8 mg/dL, we suspect low stomach acid production—a problem that adversely affects the absorption of many other nutrients. Low phosphorus can also indicate low ovarian function, liver dysfunction, or protein deficiency. People with low blood phosphorus levels are often eating too many refined sugars. We do not recommend taking phosphorus supplements, but instead encourage the consumption of naturally phosphorus-rich whole foods if levels need boosting.

High phosphorus is normal during periods of bone growth or repair. It can also indicate dysfunction of the kidneys or the parathyroid gland, which helps to regulate calcium levels and bone growth. Carbonated beverages contain unusually high levels of inorganic phosphorus, and as a result can elevate serum phosphorus levels, causing nervousness and excessive bodywide acidity.

POTASSIUM

Levels of potassium are much greater within red blood cells than outside of them. Adrenal, heart, and kidney function, as well as whole-body fluid and acid-base balance, depend upon adequate levels of this mineral.

Low potassium can reflect overactive adrenal glands, anemia, or a diet high in refined carbohydrates. People who complain of dry mouth tend to be low in potassium.

High potassium can indicate low adrenal function or kidney problems.

PROTEIN

This test provides an estimate of total protein levels in the body, based on levels of albumin and total globulin in blood serum. However, this test is not the best measure of protein intake and digestion because, if the body is deficient in protein, it can rob protein from joint capsules and muscle to keep serum protein levels in a normal range.

High protein most often is a sign of low stomach acid or underactive adrenal glands.

Low protein can point to protein malnutrition; inflammatory digestive disorders such as colitis, gastritis, or Crohn's disease; or low stomach acid.

SODIUM

Sodium is the most abundant mineral in the fluids outside of the cells, such as the blood. One of its most important functions is in regulating the

movement of fluids into and out of the cells, which affects the body's acid/
alkaline balance and adrenal, heart, and kidney function. Blood sodium
levels that are either too high or too low can be a sign of kidney disease,
dehydration, or overactive adrenal glands. Low blood sodium can mean
underactive adrenals.

HOMOCYSTEINE

Homocysteine is an amino acid that is potentially very toxic for the heart
and blood vessels. If homocysteine levels are above 8 micromoles per liter
(μmol/L) of blood, there is good chance that there are deficiencies in betaine or in one or more of the following B vitamins: vitamin B_6, vitamin
B_{12}, choline, or folic acid. Anyone under forty years old who has a family
history of heart disease or stroke should be regularly tested for homocysteine. We recommend that everyone over forty years old be given a yearly
test for homocysteine.

TABLE 4.1

Chem Screen Test Values

To help you understand the results of your own chem screen test, this table
indicates values that are considered ideal, normal, and a cause for concern.

TEST (unit of measure)	IDEAL (optimal)	REFERENCE (normal)	ALARM (needs attention)
Glucose (mg/dL)	80–100	60–110	less than 50 more than 250
Blood urea nitrogen (BUN) (mg/dL)	10–18	5–20	less than 5 more than 50
Albumin (g/dL)	4–5	3.5–5.0	less than 4

TEST (unit of measure)	IDEAL (optimal)	REFERENCE (normal)	ALARM (needs attention)
Alkaline phosphatase (ALP) (U/L)	less than 100	40–120 (may be up to 800 during times of rapid bone growth or repair)	less than 30 more than 130
Bilirubin, total (mg/dL)	0.1–1.2	0.1–1.2	more than 2.0
Bilirubin, direct (mg/dL)	0–0.2	0–0.2	more than 0.8
Bilirubin, indirect (mg/dL)	0.1–1.0	0.1–1.0	more than 1.8
Calcium (mg/dL)	9.2–10	8.2–10.2	less than 7 more than 12
Chloride (µmol/L)	100–106	97–107	less than 90 more than 115
Cholesterol, HDL (mg/dL)	more than 60	more than 55	less than 35
Cholesterol, LDL (mg/dL)	less than 100	0–130	more than 150
Carbon dioxide (CO_2) (µmol/L)	26–31	23–32	less than 18 more than 38
Creatinine (mg/dL)	0.8–1.1	0.7–1.4	more than 1.6
BUN/creatinine ratio	10–16	6–20	less than 5 more than 30
Gamma-glutamyltransferase (GGT) (U/L)	10–30	0–55 (may vary slightly in different laboratories)	more than 90

TEST (unit of measure)	IDEAL (optimal)	REFERENCE (normal)	ALARM (needs attention)
Aspartate Aminotransferase (AST) (glutamic oxaloacetic transaminase [GOT]) (U/L)	10–30	0–45 (may vary by lab)	more than 90
Alanine aminotransferase (ALT) (glutamate pyruvate transaminase [GPT]) (U/L)	10–30	0–55 (may vary by lab)	more than 90
Lactate dehydrogenase (LDH) (U/L)	140–200	100–220	less than 80 more than 240
Magnesium, serum (mg/dL)	2.0–2.7	1.6–3.5	less than 2.0 more than 3.5
Magnesium, red blood cell	——————Use laboratory reference values.——————		
Phosphorus (mg/dL)	3.0–4.0	2.5–4.5	less than 2 more than 5
Potassium (g/dL)	4.0–4.5	3.5–5.3	less than 3 more than 6
Protein (g/dL)	6.9–7.4	6.0–8.0	less than 5.9 more than 8.5
Sodium (μmol/L)	135–142	135–145	less than 125 more than 155

Signs and Symptoms
of Low Adrenal Function

Some of the results of the chem panel can point to problems with adrenal function. The chronic fatigue many women experience postpartum is often related to adrenal glands that were tapped out during pregnancy and birth. The following is a list of symptoms that may indicate tired adrenals:

- A bout of cold or flu followed by chronic fatigue.
- Chemical sensitivities.
- Chronic fatigue.
- Cravings for salt or other foods.
- Dizziness.
- Extreme fatigue following exercise.
- Failure to sweat during exercise.
- Food sensitivities.
- Low systolic blood pressure (the systolic pressure is the first number in a blood-pressure reading; for example, the 130 in a blood pressure of 130/90).
- Standing blood pressure lower than reclining blood pressure.
- Respiratory distress.
- Sparse body hair, especially on the arms and legs.

If a woman is experiencing many of these symptoms and her chem panel results point us toward adrenal exhaustion, we usually do a reproductive and adrenal hormone test to further pinpoint the problem. (More about the adrenal hormones, tests that measure their activity, and what you can do to help these glands bounce back after pregnancy appears in Chapter 9.)

Variations on the Chem Screen Theme

As noted earlier, the individual tests given as part of a chem screen may vary, depending on physician or laboratory. Some chem panels include tests to measure immune function, levels of certain hormones, blood clotting time, or other variables. In some instances, the tests we discuss later in this chapter—separately from the chem screen—will be included.

Depending on the results of the chem panel, and on an individual's symptoms, one or more other tests may be ordered to identify where she needs nutritional, hormonal, or lifestyle support. If symptoms point strongly to the need for other tests, these can be ordered along with the chem panel, either at the initial visit or at a later one. As you read through the chapters to come, you should be able to do some of your own detective work to determine which tests might be most helpful for you.

Urinary Organic Acid Analysis

Organic acids are a broad class of compounds required for the fundamental metabolic processes of the body. The urinary organic acid analysis has traditionally been used to identify severe inborn metabolic problems that are fatal in early childhood, but a number of the organic acid compounds measured with this test have proven clinically useful in detecting nutritional deficiencies in adults.

Elevation of specific organic acids can indicate blocks or disorders in important metabolic pathways. A trained eye can look at the results of an organic acid analysis and see impairments or deficiencies in nutrients necessary for fatty acid metabolism, carbohydrate metabolism, and energy production. This test can also yield valuable information about the body's levels of nutritional cofactors needed for the manufacture of neurotransmitter molecules and for liver detoxification. We can even find markers that reveal whether a patient has intestinal parasites or other infections using this test.

Comprehensive Detoxification Profile

The liver's ability to neutralize and eliminate environmental toxins, those created by normal digestive activity, and "used-up" hormones and immune factors, has a much greater bearing on health than conventional medicine would have you believe. The comprehensive detoxification profile is a laboratory test that gives information about both your exposure to these substances and your liver's ability to handle the load.

As we saw in the preceding chapter, each phase and pathway of liver detoxification requires specific nutrients to run smoothly. Any deficiency of these nutrients will result in an increase in toxic burden, which may in turn contribute to chronic fatigue, environmental illness, allergies, fibromyalgia, inflammatory joint disease, and other chronic ailments. The comprehensive detoxification profile assesses the demand for and the availability of these nutrients. This test entails ingesting aspirin, acetaminophen, and caffeine, and then giving both urine and blood samples for analysis to determine how well the major liver detoxification pathways required to detoxify these substance are functioning and what nutritional support may be needed for optimal liver function. If test results point to a severe problem, a referral to a liver specialist may be called for.

For a sample of a comprehensive detoxification profile, see page 277.

Other Tests

There are a number of laboratory tests that can be useful for diagnostic purposes as well. Essential fatty acid analysis, serum lipid peroxide testing, antioxidant analysis, mineral analysis, amino acid analysis, intestinal permeability testing, and hormone testing all contribute key information to the functional nutrition practitioner's healing quest. Other commonly used tests check for insulin resistance, brain neurotransmitter balance, food allergies, and the more sophisticated inflammatory chemicals that can affect the heart and vascular system, such as the apolipoproteins A and B (apoA and apoB), sensitive C-reactive protein, and fibrinogen. A complete patient history and examination should guide the doctor in choosing the appropriate tests for each individual.

Choosing Your Health-Care Team

If the diet and lifestyle changes and supplemental nutrients recommended in this book do not bring your body back into a balance that feels right to you, we highly recommend consulting with a doctor who is familiar with functional medicine tests and the methods for interpreting them that we describe in these pages.

In the Resources section at the back of this book, you will find a list of organizations that educate doctors to be good nutritionists. Most of the doctors who have trained with these organizations can be expected to be familiar with the tests described throughout this book. There is also a list of laboratories that run these tests. Some of them may allow you to order the supplies and information you need to do the tests yourself, by mail. If you cannot locate a good nutritional or functional medicine doctor in or near your town, you can use mail-order tests and contact an organization that can help you interpret test results. These organizations, also listed under Mail-Order Lab Tests in the Resources section, will supply you with practical recommendations you can implement based on the results of your lab tests.

Now that we have seen how important your body's nutritional reserves are to your health and have looked at some of the laboratory tests that can help identify many of your own specific nutritional deficiencies, let us look at some of the ways that you can begin to replenish your postpartum nutrient deficiencies. The recommendations we offer can help even if you are years or decades postpartum. It is important to rebuild your nutrient reserves for your own well-being. It is even more important to do this if you are planning to have more children. In the following two chapters, we will show you how you can replenish your postpartum nutritional reserves through diet and nutritional supplementation.

5

Building Nutrient
Reserves with Diet

One of the classic medical textbooks on obstetrics, an imposing volume titled *Williams Obstetrics* (McGraw-Hill, 2001), devotes only three of more than sixteen hundred pages to the postpartum period. This makes sense in light of the fact that the average obstetrician (OB) does not participate much in postpartum care. For an uncomplicated birth, the OB shows up as the baby is emerging and zooms off as soon as he or she knows all is well.

Even if the OB were available to answer questions about how to eat during the postpartum months, he or she might not have much information to offer you. In those three pages on postpartum care in *Williams Obstetrics,* the only dietary advice the authors give is that women who have just given birth need not observe any dietary restrictions, and that they should eat an "appetizing general diet." Some women might find fried chicken, soda pop, and doughnuts to be the most appetizing foods around, but we know that these foods do not give a new mother's body the nutritional support it needs—and that nutrients drawn from her already depleted stores will be needed to process those foods, leaving her with an even greater deficit. Women need more specific information about how to nourish their bodies during postpartum recovery and breastfeeding. Advice on the ideal diet during pregnancy is easy to find in the average bookstore. It is much harder to find the facts on what to eat postpartum.

When you are engaged in baby care, putting nutritional advice into practice can be a formidable challenge. Some mothers give up on food preparation completely during the first months of their babies' lives, subsisting on takeout or ready-made packaged meals that do not meet their nutritional needs. However, it is important to eat nourishing, nutrient-replenishing foods during the pregnancy-recovery period to give yourself the best opportunity to avoid long-term nutrient deficiencies that may cause serious disease later on in life. In this chapter, we will guide you on how to eat to replenish your tapped-out nutrient stores, but will also pass on some tips that will help you to make nourishing meals quickly and easily at home.

Your Pregnancy Diet: How Did You Do?

Some women go overboard during pregnancy, eating as much as they like of whatever they like. These are the women who say, "It's fine for me to eat this entire jumbo-sized chocolate bar—I'm craving it, so my body must need it!" If this were really true, we would all have intense cravings for broccoli or Brussels sprouts or kale rather than for cake, potato chips, or ice cream. When you crave sugary or fatty junk food, it is usually because your body is lacking an important nutrient. For some people, eating junk food is also a way to numb the emotions.

Of course, some women do crave healthy foods during pregnancy. Sour apples or lemons, red meat, and peaches are a few examples of common cravings that probably indicate a need for the nutrients these foods contain. Acidic, vitamin C–rich fruits help your body to absorb iron; red meat is an excellent source of iron and essential amino acids and is often craved by even avowed vegetarians during pregnancy; and peaches are a very rich source of beta-carotene.

While women who eat with abandon during pregnancy have a better

Patty's Story

Patty felt terrible for six months after her son's birth. She was forty-five pounds overweight and felt completely exhausted. Still, she found the energy to propel herself and her husband along on a terrible emotional roller-coaster ride. She constantly felt afraid that she was an unfit mother, that her baby would be taken away from her because she couldn't handle motherhood.

When she went for prenatal care, her obstetrician told her to eat pretty much anything she wanted, whenever she wanted, and to drink a canned meal-replacement drink once a day to make sure she was getting the recommended daily allowance (RDA) of all the vitamins and minerals. She thought that by eating whatever she wanted, she was listening to her body.

She had never really eaten vegetables and liked only a few kinds of fruit, and that didn't change while she was pregnant. Instead, she devoured all kinds of candy, ice cream, french fries, cookies, cake, pasta, and sodas. Her mother's mashed potatoes were as close as Patty got to health food. The pregnancy books she read said to get plenty of protein, and she thought it was okay to get hers from fried chicken, hot dogs, and fast-food hamburgers. The more sugar she ate, the more sugar she craved. She thought that the nutrition drink would make up for whatever she was missing.

A friend referred Patty to me after her own doctor told her, "It's just a little postpartum depression." She just knew there had to be more to it than that, and was ready to do something more proactive than swallowing some Prozac. She felt like the time had come for her to take control of her health—that she owed it to her baby, her husband, and herself. Both breast cancer and heart disease run in her family, and she said she knew that her diet from this point on would influence whether or not she would live to see her son graduate from college.

I first ran a chem screen blood test. When the results came back, I told Patty she had slightly high fasting blood glucose, high triglycerides, and high LDL cholesterol. Two of her liver enzyme tests were moderately high, and her thyroid gland function was borderline low. I then measured her blood sugar and insulin levels before and after having her drink some very sugary water. This revealed that she was insulin resistant—the levels of insulin and sugars in her bloodstream were too high. This is a prediabetic condition that can be corrected with a good diet and supplements, and I felt that doing so would fix a lot of Patty's problems. I also told her that she needed to put her son in a stroller and start walking daily for exercise, and to slowly increase the length and pace of their walks.

I recommended that she start eating more foods high in fiber, like whole beans and grains, fresh fruits, and vegetables. These foods can actually lower high blood sugars and insulin levels. For protein, she learned to enjoy fresh fish, lean meat, and chicken and turkey. I also designed a customized amino acid powder for Patty, based on her blood amino acid profile. These measures helped to control her moods and lessened her cravings for sweets and white bread, which she was to stay away from.

Patty asked me if she had to stop eating fat to lose the weight she had gained. I explained to her the importance of the good fats, like the omega-3 oils and gamma-linolenic acid (GLA). I joked that what she needed was an "oil change," because the fats and sugars she was eating were affecting the way her cells responded to insulin and other hormones. I advised her to cut out most red meat, fried food, and dairy products for a while, and to take fish oil and black currant seed oil supplements, as well as 200 micrograms of the mineral chromium three times a day. Soon she found she had the energy to exercise again and enjoyed taking her baby for long walks in his stroller.

Within three weeks, Patty said she was feeling much better. Her energy was back, and as her blood sugar stabilized, so did her moods. Eventually she got back to her normal weight and she continues to feel well on her diet. She gives herself the occasional sweet treat, but says that she notices a tendency to crave sugar for days afterward, a situation that taking the amino acid powder and chromium helps to correct. All in all, she says, limiting sugar intake is a small price to pay for feeling great and being able to maintain her normal weight again. In retrospect, she says she sees that the problems she experienced could have been avoided if she had known how to nourish her body during her pregnancy—and she is greatly relieved that her son is doing fine in spite of the way she ate while she was pregnant with him.

—D.R.

chance of getting everything they and their babies need simply because they are taking in larger servings of a wider variety of foods, they often get too many *anti*nutrients ("bad" fats, additives, and sugar) and not enough of the nutrients their bodies really need to build a baby. They may end up overweight yet undernourished.

Other women go to the opposite extreme, eating exactly what they believe to be the ideal pregnancy diet, restricting calories to control their weight gain, and valiantly fighting off their worst cravings or finding "acceptable" substitutes (which, according to many sources, means finding low-fat or nonfat versions of fatty foods). If women follow the typical guidelines, they will probably get good enough nutrition to have a healthy pregnancy and a healthy baby, but chances are good that they will have some sort of significant deficit postpartum. The ideal pregnancy diet falls somewhere between these two extremes.

What about pregnancy weight gain? How much is too much? This varies from person to person. A woman who is very thin when she becomes pregnant might gain more than a woman who is heavier to begin with, and she may need that extra fat for breastfeeding. Your doctor or midwife should be able to tell whether your weight gain is excessive. It is highly unlikely, however, that you will gain too much weight as long as you eat according to the guidelines in this chapter—they can be used prenatally as well as postpartum.

Mothers who opt for a low-fat diet—20 percent or less of calories from fat—in an effort to stave off excessive weight gain or to be healthier at any point during pregnancy are risking toxemia, growth problems, behavioral or neurological problems, and prematurity in their babies. Why? Because a diet low in fat is also low in the essential fatty acids that support the development of the baby's nervous system and the continued health of the mother's nervous system. As you will see later in this chapter, essential fats also support a healthy pregnancy and a timely birth in more ways than you might expect. The typical low-fat diet is also lacking in the amino acids your body needs to build your baby's tissues, and tends to include too many processed foods made from sugar and flour.

The "Food Tree" Plan

Ideally, new parents should have a "food tree" in place before the birth of their child. A few weeks before your due date, ask a friend or family member to enlist several people to provide your family with home-cooked evening meals every day during the first postpartum weeks. Have this individual friend emphasize that the food tree is not about socializing—those who bring the meal should stay for only a few minutes, and then quietly slip off so that you and your partner don't feel obliged to entertain them. Also, let your friend or relative know what kinds of food you want to eat in those first postpartum weeks—or give him or her a copy of this book with the diet guidelines marked! Then the food tree participants will be more likely to bring you the foods your body really needs to replenish itself.

Immediately Postpartum

From what we have heard, there is very little to compare to the first meal that comes after a long, hard labor and birth. Have whatever you like. Drink plenty of water and (preferably fresh-squeezed) juices to begin replenishing your body. Try to incorporate the fish soup with seaweed that Chinese women use. It is loaded with minerals and vitamins. (For a simple recipe, see page 91.)

One woman we know requested and devoured a huge platter of sushi soon after she gave birth to her daughter. Fresh, raw salmon, mackerel, and yellowtail are excellent sources of docosahexaenoic acid (DHA) and eicosapentaenoic acid (EPA)—a good start for a new mother and her baby! If sushi is the type of meal you choose, make sure to eat the pickled ginger and wasabi horseradish that come with it. They will help to kill any bacteria that the raw fish may contain.

Fish Soup with Seaweed

BASIC RECIPE

⅓ package (1.76 ounces) hiziki-type seaweed
⅓ package (1.76 ounces) kombu-type seaweed
2 large carrots, preferably organic, raw (unpeeled)
2 scallions, raw
¼ cup snow peas
¼ cup fresh cilantro
2 cans (14.5 ounces each) organic chicken broth
  (such as Shelton's)
½ pound fresh salmon

1. Place the seaweed in a bowl and add just enough water to cover it. Allow it to soak for twenty to thirty minutes.
2. While the seaweed is soaking, chop the carrots, scallions, snow peas, and cilantro into bite-sized pieces, and place them in a sturdy 4-quart cooking pot.
3. Cut the salmon into cubes and add them to the pot.
4. Add the chicken broth to the pot.
5. Add the soaked seaweed. Allow all the ingredients to sit for twenty to thirty minutes.
6. Gradually bring the mixture to a simmer over low heat, and allow it to simmer for twenty minutes or until the vegetables are tender. Serve hot.

You can find seaweed in Asian markets and at many health food stores. Emerald Cove brand kombu and hijiki are good products that are relatively easy to find.

VARIATIONS

1. If you prefer, you can substitute a total of 2½ cups of any chopped vegetable or vegetables of your choice for the carrots, cilantro, scallions, and snow peas. Other good choices include celery, red peppers, and zucchini.

2. To make the soup with a miso broth, substitute 3 cups of water for the chicken broth and cook as directed. Immediately before-serving, mix 2 heaping tablespoons of miso paste with a little water and stir until smooth. Remove the pot from the heat and add the miso paste mixture, stirring until blended. (You should never boil miso, as it will curdle.) Most miso is made of fermented soybeans; however, for this recipe, you can use chickpea or rice miso as well.

3. If you wish, you can substitute an equal amount of any other type of fatty fish, such as fresh cod, mackerel, or tuna, for the salmon.

Dietary Tips for Nursing Mothers

Significant hormonal shifts go on in your body when your milk comes in for the first time, and this is often compounded by difficulties in establishing a nursing routine. Midwives jokingly refer to the forgetfulness and moodiness many new mothers experience as "milk-brain." Some women become weepy during this time. Be patient and expect the nursing relationship to take a few weeks to establish.

Avoid acidic and gas-producing foods for the first few weeks postpartum. Colic—inconsolable crying that can last for hours at a time—has been linked to gastrointestinal distress, and often responds well to the elimination of certain foods from the nursing mother's diet. To be on the safe side, avoid all of the following in the first month to three months of your baby's life:

- Alcohol.
- Brewer's yeast.
- Carbonated beverages.
- Chocolate and other caffeine-containing foods.
- Most dairy products and other foods containing lactose (milk sugar). Hard cheeses, butter, and yogurt with live cultures have

very little to no lactose, and should be all right as long as you are not allergic to the milk protein casein.

- Gas-forming vegetables (broccoli, Brussels sprouts, cabbage, cauliflower, and the like).
- Oranges and orange juice.
- Strawberries.

After those initial weeks, you can try having these foods again, one at a time, to see if your baby reacts to them. Add only one food back every two or three days so that you can discern your baby's reaction easily. If he becomes colicky or develops a skin rash or redness around his anus, he may have a sensitivity to the food. If that happens, wait a few more weeks before trying it again. By the time your baby is about three months old, his digestive system should be mature enough to deal with most of the foods you eat. However, acidic fruits such as oranges and strawberries could cause your baby to develop rashes for as long as he is nursing. If your baby is colicky in spite of your having eliminated all the above foods, try eliminating all grains except rice for a week to see if that helps. Some babies react to foods that contain gluten, a protein found in wheat, oats, rye, amaranth, and spelt.

A sad truth is that mother's milk is laced with the chemicals that all human beings are exposed to. Dioxins and other chemicals are stored in fatty breast tissue and enter your baby's body when she nurses. While this is a terrible fact of life for the new mother to face, it should not change your mind about breastfeeding. Breast milk is still the perfect food for babies, and no formula manufacturer can match it.

If you need to boost your milk production, try an old folk remedy that many European women still use: Go to a pub and order up a pint of the darkest beer they have. (Or have your partner bring home a six-pack.) No one really knows exactly why beer helps with nursing, but many mothers will attest to its effectiveness—and as long as you have only *one* beer, a nursing baby should not be harmed by the alcohol it contains. Herbs such as goat's rue and blessed thistle also help increase milk production. Deep green leafy vegetables can support increased milk production as well. If these veggies don't agree with your baby, try taking small amounts of concentrated sources of green nutrients such as chlorella or liquid chlorophyll.

Diet, Breastfeeding, and Weight Loss

The average mother loses about ten to twenty pounds the first four weeks postpartum, then about one and a half pounds a month in the span of the next four to six months. Contrary to popular belief, not all research shows a difference between nursing and bottle-feeding mothers when it comes to weight loss. Women are often told that they will lose their pregnancy weight faster if they nurse, but some studies show that nursing mothers actually hold on to excess weight a bit longer, because they need that extra five or so pounds to make sufficient milk for their babies.

Nursing mothers need about 500 extra calories a day. If you follow the postpartum guidelines supplied in the rest of this chapter, your body will tell you how much to eat and what foods to include. You won't need to count calories or measure out servings to ensure that your baby is getting what he needs and that your nutrient stores are being built back up. Don't try to decrease your fat intake, but do pay attention to the *type* of fat you are eating.

The Basic Postpartum Diet

The basic postpartum diet is a simple but healthy and wholesome one. It can best be summed up by the following guidelines:

- Eat foods that supply your body with essential fatty acids, like fresh salmon, nuts, and seeds.
- Eat whole, preferably organic, foods—whole grains, fresh vegetables and fruits, unprocessed meats, nuts, and seeds, for example.
- Avoid refined sugars and flour, during pregnancy and postpartum.
- Eat foods that supply your body with antioxidants (mainly fresh fruits and vegetables).

Melody's Story

Within days of giving birth to her daughter, Melody was thinking of herself as a bad mother. Every night at about five P.M., Skye would begin to cry inconsolably, and she wouldn't stop until after eight P.M., when she would pass out from sheer exhaustion. Melody and her partner tried everything they could think of to soothe the baby, who wouldn't nurse during these episodes. They bounced her, rocked her, sang to her, walked her, bathed her, danced with her, and massaged her belly. Sometimes they would manage to calm her for a few minutes, but it was almost as if the baby was determined to stick to her crying schedule, come what may. Melody and her partner were frustrated and exhausted.

Melody cut out the foods her lactation consultant suggested, and that helped a little bit. Then, a friend recommended a book called *The Aware Baby* by Aletha J. Solter, which talked about how babies sometimes need to cry, and that if you make sure all their basic needs are met—they are fed, dry, and not too cold or too hot, and you are giving them the physical contact they need—and they still want to cry, they may be discharging some kind of trauma or frustration that could have happened before birth, during birth, or after. Skye's birth was pretty traumatic; Melody had been in labor for almost forty hours and ended up having an emergency C-section.

The book recommended that you just hold your baby close and let her cry if she needs to, and don't react as if crying is wrong or bad—let her know you love her and accept her whether she is crying or happy. As soon as they changed their attitudes about Skye's crying, Melody says—they just held her tight, let her howl, and told her she was doing just fine and they loved her—the episodes became shorter and she would go in and out of the crying spontaneously, not in response to anything they were doing. Melody found herself crying right along with Skye sometimes, and she says she thinks it helped her to let go of some of the trauma she had had with the birth and with being a new mom. After the baby finished crying, rather than falling asleep, she would become relaxed and alert for a while, and then she'd nurse herself to sleep

The nightly crying continued until Skye was about two months old, but when Melody and her partner reframed it as a positive thing for her instead of something they were bad parents for being unable to stop, it all began to seem okay. Now Skye is thirteen months old, and Melody says she still seems to need to let loose and have a good cry now and then.

- Eat slowly and chew your food thoroughly.
- Eat a source of nutrient-laden fiber, such as ground flaxseeds.

EAT FOODS THAT SUPPLY YOUR BODY
WITH ESSENTIAL FATTY ACIDS

Fatty acids are the final breakdown product of fats in the diet—the part of the fats you eat that is either stored or used in the cells for energy. Fatty acids were once viewed as nothing more than a source of stored calories, but modern research has shown that the quality of fatty acids in the body has profound effects on human health. Diseases related to inflammation, hormone imbalances, the immune system, behavioral problems, and the heart can often be partially or completely resolved if essential fatty acid levels are balanced through dietary changes or supplementation.

Omega-3 Fatty Acids

When you are pregnant, the developing fetus requires large amounts of two specific fatty acids, arachidonic acid (AA) and docosahexaenoic acid (DHA), to build brain and nerve cell membranes. Once a baby reaches about six months of age, his or her body will be able to make DHA and AA from other fatty acids, but while still in utero and in the first six months of life, these fats must be supplied in exact form by the mother's body—first through the placenta, then through breast milk. More than half of the nerve connections in baby's brain form during the first year of life, and the integrity of these connections is dependent upon the fatty acid supply from the mother. Ideally, mother's milk supplies DHA and AA to her baby through nursing for at least a year.

In Chapter 3, you saw how the fats you eat are transformed into hormonelike messenger molecules called prostaglandins, and how the balance of essential fats in your diet dictates the balance of prostaglandins in your body. These fats are also needed for proper brain and nervous system function in people of all ages, but are needed more than ever during gestation and in your baby's infancy, when those systems are undergoing their fastest period of growth.

The omega-3 fat docosahexaenoic acid, or DHA, is the most important structural and cognitive (brain-function–related) fat for your brain and for your baby's brain. The placenta draws DHA from the mother's body like a vacuum cleaner, and the milk ducts continue to drain her stores for as long as her baby nurses. If you do not keep replenishing your supply, your emotional and physical well-being will most likely be compromised in the postpartum period and beyond.

The research of Dr. Joseph Hibbeln, a psychiatrist, lipid biologist, and senior clinical investigator with the Section of Nutritional Neuroscience at the National Institute on Alcohol and Alcohol Abuse's Laboratory of Membrane Biochemistry and Biophysics, beautifully illustrates the connection between omega-3 lack and postpartum depression. Dr. Hibbeln examined fish consumption and the incidence of postpartum depression (PPD) in several countries, and found that the more fish women ate, the less likely they were to develop PPD.

Other research has shown that with each successive pregnancy, blood levels of DHA fall further, and that this dramatically increases a woman's risk of pregnancy complications. This is why it is especially important to build up your reserves of these good oils if you are thinking of having another child. Pregnant mothers with the lowest levels of DHA and eicosapentaenoic acid (EPA), another important fatty acid, in their red blood cells are nearly eight times more likely to develop preeclampsia, a complication of pregnancy characterized by elevated blood pressure, than are women with the highest levels of DHA and EPA.

Vegetarian women tend to have much lower levels of DHA than nonvegetarians, and may have more pregnancy complications because of this deficiency. Women who are deficient in EPA and DHA have a sixfold greater risk of developing serious mental disorders such as depression and obsessive-compulsive disorder, and this risk remains higher for two years after giving birth. Vegetarian mothers can get DHA from some of the algae-based products designed with them in mind.

Babies and toddlers score higher on tests of intelligence and visual acuity if their mothers ate fish a few times weekly during pregnancy. Breastfed babies, who get a lot more DHA from mother's milk than their bottle-fed counterparts get from formula, also do better on intelligence and vision tests, and they are less vulnerable to attention deficit disorders and other behavioral and learning problems.

If you eat the typical Western diet, you were probably already depleted of DHA and EPA when you became pregnant. Your baby's body drew on your omega-3 stores to build its brain, nervous system, and cell membranes, and left you even more depleted. There is good scientific evidence that a lack of omega-3 fats passes from generation to generation; if your mother did not pass much on to you, your body has fewer stores to draw from during your own pregnancy, and if you have a daughter, her body could have even less of these essential fats to fortify her own offspring. It is therefore essential to replenish your omega-3 reserves.

Fish is the best natural source of DHA. Not all fish are good sources of this fatty acid and EPA. Fish that live in deep, cold waters, such as salmon, cod, sardines, anchovies, albacore tuna, herring, and mackerel, are your best sources of these essential fats. Because fish, like every other creature on the planet, contain toxins that come from the foods they eat, limit fish consumption to three times a week. Avoid swordfish, shark, and tilefish entirely when you are pregnant or nursing, because these species tend to retain higher levels of toxins in their flesh. Some nutritionists recommend farmed fish over wild fish to avoid toxins, but farmed fish are generally fed foods high in unsaturated oils such as soy and corn, so their DHA levels are lower. The best answer is probably to try to vary the type of fish you eat, alternating between farm-raised and wild-caught fish.

We recommend eating high-DHA omega-3 eggs. These eggs are laid by chickens fed a vegetarian, DHA-rich diet with algae added to their food. They are a great source of this essential fat, especially for women who don't like fish. (Although we are not aware of any studies on the intelligence and visual acuity of the chickens that lay omega-3 eggs, it is likely that they and their offspring are sharper than the average clucker!) Omega-3 eggs also contain six times more of the antioxidant vitamin E than other eggs.

We also recommend taking EFA supplements throughout pregnancy, nursing, and beyond. We will tell you how to choose them in the next chapter.

Flaxseed oil, which is high in another omega-3 fatty acid, alpha-linolenic acid (ALA), is widely touted as an ideal omega-3 supplement for those who would rather not eat fish. ALA is indeed similar in structure to DHA and EPA, but the ALA molecule is slightly shorter in length—causing it to be termed a short-chain omega-3—than these other two long-chain omega-3s. Thus, in order for ALA to be made into "good" prostaglandins or to build nervous-system tissues and cell membranes that function optimally, it must be transformed into EPA or DHA. Some research shows that this transformation can fulfill the body's EPA and DHA needs adequately, while other research casts doubt upon the body's ability to transform enough ALA to meet its needs.

The scientific jury is still out on this one, but after looking at hundreds of blood tests for fatty acid levels, we feel the best way to ensure that your DHA and EPA levels are sufficient is to eat foods that contain DHA and EPA. If you want a vegetarian supplement of these oils, seek out the ones made from algae. That is where the fish get their long-chain omega-3s. ALA can be a valuable addition to the diet, helping to balance out skewed omega-3 to omega-6 ratios.

We do not recommend that you use a lot of flaxseed *oil* to supply your diet with ALA. (We will discuss the use of flaxseeds themselves a little later in this chapter.) Flaxseed oil is one the least stable oils known. In other words, it spoils easily and goes rancid. If you eat rancid oil, you are ingesting toxic free radicals that have to be soaked up by your antioxidant stores, leaving fewer antioxidants to control the rest of the free radicals that are constantly forming throughout your body. Walnuts and pumpkinseeds are other good sources of ALA.

Omega-6 Fatty Acids

When I told Patty that she needed an "oil change," (see Patty's Story on page 87), I meant that her unbalanced consumption of certain fats and oils—saturated fats from fried meats and desserts, and chips and fries cooked in hydrogenated omega-6 oils—had affected the ability of her body to make energy at the cellular level. Omega-6 fats have a different structure from the omega-3s, and when they are incorporated into cell membranes, they subtly alter the membrane's structure and activity.

It is true that mother's milk is the best source of omega-3s for babies, but the amount of these EFAs in breast milk varies widely depending on the mother's diet. Inuit women, who eat fish and seal meat daily, have a ratio of omega-6 to long-chain omega-3 fats (EPA and DHA) of about 4:1. At the same time, one study showed that the average American woman's milk contains these fats in a ratio of *175:1!* If the omega-6/omega-3 ratio becomes skewed in this way, an imbalance of prostaglandin production results, increasing your vulnerability to allergies, autoimmune diseases, mood disorders, joint pain, and other problems. By cutting down on omega-6 fats—in particular, linoleic acid from processed vegetable, nut, and seed oils—and boosting your intake of omega-3s, you can supply your baby and yourself with a more ideal ratio of these fats.

Corn oil, soybean oil, safflower oil, sunflower oil, and cottonseed oil all contain plentiful amounts of linoleic acid (LA), one of the omega-6 fats. These oils are found in a great many processed foods, and it is the rare Westerner who does not get plenty of linoleic acid every day. Worse, these oils are usually hydrogenated or partially hydrogenated to make them solid instead of liquid. This process alters the molecular composition of the fatty acids so that they are inflexible. Over time, these inflexible fats are incorporated into cell membranes, compromising the cells' ability to bring in needed substances and flush out wastes. Hydrogenated fats also contribute to an increasing burden of "bad" prostaglandins. The fatty acids in hydrogenated oils are known as *trans fats* or *trans-fatty acids,* and they pass right into your breast milk and into your baby's body. Read labels carefully; if you see the words *hydrogenated* or *partially hydrogenated* on a label, put the product back on the shelf. Be forewarned: You will find hydrogenated and partially hydrogenated oils in just about every type of processed food, including cookies, crackers, frozen foods, margarine, potato and corn chips, pies, pastries, salad dressings, and soups.

It is unlikely that your health will be improved if you add more foods containing linoleic acid to your diet. Supplemental black currant seed, borage, and evening primrose seed oils, however, contain a specific omega-6 fat, gamma-linolenic acid (GLA), that is scarce in food. The most significant food source of GLA is oatmeal. This fat has been demonstrated to be helpful for relief from attention deficit disorder, multiple sclerosis, depression, and mood swings. GLA can be transformed in the body into an anti-inflammatory, brain-supporting prostaglandin called prostaglandin E_1 (PGE_1). (We will talk more about these beneficial omega-6 fats in the next chapter.)

Essential Fatty Acid Analysis

The essential fatty acid analysis is one of the most useful tests of nutritional status. It gives a clear picture of the amounts and ratios of many key fats found in an individual's blood and tissues.

No doubt you can see why we favor evaluating the fatty acid reserves of any woman who is pregnant or is contemplating pregnancy, and why we often do so postpartum. In fact, the majority of patients we see have significant fatty-acid imbalances. This is largely due to the widespread use of vegetable oils in cooking, as well as the processing of oils to eliminate or reduce the amount of easily spoiled, stronger-tasting omega-3s. Most of our patients are notably deficient in the omega-3 fats DHA, EPA, ALA, and GLA, and have too much of other, less healthy, more inflammatory saturated and omega-6 polyunsaturated fatty acids (like arachidonic acid, or AA) in their blood and tissues. When the levels of all of these types of fats are brought into balance, both through diet and the use of supplements, many patients experience relief from pain, depression, and mood swings.

EAT WHOLE, PREFERABLY ORGANIC, FOODS

To ensure that you are getting plenty of the nutrients that help build your baby's body and maintain your own health, eat a well-rounded whole foods diet throughout pregnancy and postpartum. Whole foods have undergone little or no processing before they arrive on your plate; they are as close as possible to the way nature made them. In general, whole foods are found around the outer edges of the supermarket—fresh fruits and vegetables, bulk foods, some dairy foods (those that have undergone the least processing, such as butter, soft and hard cheeses, and unsweetened yogurt), and meats are whole foods. Whole foods do not contain "empty calories." Every calorie is accompanied by vitamins, minerals, and other important nutrients. During pregnancy and nursing, you are indeed eating for two, and the more nutrient-dense and wholesome your diet is, the healthier you and your baby will be.

If a food comes in a package and the label lists ingredients you do not immediately recognize, it isn't a whole food. The presence of added preservatives, dyes, sugars, flavorings, and oils generally means that something has been processed enough to require extra flavor or improved texture or color. Artificial preservatives generally mean that the natural preservatives—antioxidant vitamins—have been processed out. It is fine to use some time-savers, such as canned beans and frozen vegetables, but generally, the fresher your food is, the better.

Become a label-reader. If you need an advanced degree in chemistry to decipher the label on a food product, put it back on the shelf. Do you like strawberry ice cream? On the label of one brand we looked at, we found forty-three ingredients, including substances called amyl acetate, benzyl isobutyrate, butyric acid, cinnamyl isobutyrate, cinnamyl valerate, cognac essential oil, diacetyl, dipropyl ketone, ethyl butyrate, ethyl cinnamate, and ethyl heptanoate. And you thought all you needed to make strawberry ice cream was cream, strawberries, and sugar!

The truth about food additives such as artificial flavorings is that, in most cases, we do not know whether these ingredients can cause harm or how they interact with one another in the body. There are hundreds of additives that are commonly used in processed foods. However, when their safety is evaluated, they are studied individually (in rodents, not in humans) and for no longer than two years at a time. Such tests cannot possibly take into account how all of these chemicals interact in the human body over a lifetime of use. Neither do they take into account how they might change during the cooking or further processing of foods that contain them. If you would rather be safe than sorry, it makes sense to minimize the amounts of such substances present in your diet.

When you eat meat, eggs, or dairy products, choose organic, free-range varieties. These are more nutritious because the animals that produced them are better nourished, and they are relatively free of the pesticides, antibiotics, and hormones that contaminate conventionally raised varieties of these foods. Wild fish and game and range-fed livestock, which have fed on omega-3 rich plants, are much higher in the important omega-3 fatty acids than are conventional, farm-raised fish or grain-fed livestock.

You are also much better off with organic vegetables and grains. They taste better and are more nutrient-dense because they are grown in healthier soil that is richer in minerals. If for some reason you cannot purchase the organic versions of all types of foods, however, it is more important to buy organically produced animal-based foods. Toxins are much more highly concentrated in these than in plant foods.

AVOID REFINED SUGARS AND FLOUR

Women who are able to dramatically reduce their consumption of refined sugars and flour find that their mood swings even out and their excess weight comes off. Not only will this shift in eating habits create room in your diet for whole foods—especially vegetables—but it will go a long way toward establishing blood-sugar and insulin balance.

All pregnant women tend to become slightly *insulin resistant*. Insulin is a hormone that carries sugar into the body's cells to be burned for energy. Insulin resistance means that the cells no longer heed insulin's message as well as they once did. When insulin resistance sets in, the body begins to boost insulin production to try to force the cells to hear its message and respond. As the insides of the cells clamor for energy in the form of blood sugar, more and more insulin is released to try to meet their needs. You might compare this to trying to talk to your normally sensitive and receptive partner while he is watching a favorite program on television—you may have to yell or put your body between him and the TV set in order to get your message across. Similarly, your body turns up the "volume" by increasing its production of insulin. This may get the message across for a while, but if you do not change your diet, it will not work for long. Insulin resistance can be the root cause of the deep fatigue many women, like Patty, feel postpartum. (See Patty's Story on page 87.)

While many women's levels of blood sugar and insulin ultimately return to normal after they give birth, some pregnant women go on to develop gestational diabetes, and some continue to be insulin resistant postpartum.

Others are never diagnosed with gestational diabetes, but do have subtle, ongoing blood sugar imbalances postpartum. This is what happened to Patty, and correcting the problem with dietary changes did wonders for her health.

Whenever you eat foods containing carbohydrates—groups of sugar molecules bound together by chemical bonds—your pancreas, a small organ located near the opening of your small intestines, releases insulin into the bloodstream. Eating lots of rapidly digested carbohydrates stimulates a strong, quick release of insulin, while eating moderate amounts of slowly digested carbohydrates stimulates a gradual, moderate insulin release. Carbohydrates that have had much of the fiber, oils, and nutrients processed out are referred to as *simple* (or *refined*) *carbohydrates*. Those that are closer to the form in which nature made them are *complex* (or *unrefined*) *carbohydrates*. The simpler the carbohydrate, the faster it is digested, and the stronger the insulin response it elicits.

The carbohydrates found in whole grains are complex. A wheat berry, for example, is a source of complex carbohydrates and is a whole food. So is brown rice. Your digestive tract has to process the fiber, protein, and essential fats that package the carbohydrates in these foods. Then enzymes dissolve the bonds between the sugar molecules so that they can be absorbed into your bloodstream through the wall of your small intestines and used as cellular fuel. The absorption of carbohydrates from whole foods is gradual, and so is the rise in blood sugar and insulin that follows.

Refined Sugar

Sucrose, or table sugar, is a simple carbohydrate. Simple carbohydrates are, in essence, predigested—processing has removed most of the components of the food as it is found in nature, just as your digestive tract is designed to do. This allows the carbohydrates to break down into sugars almost immediately, and to pass right into your bloodstream with little additional processing by the enzymes in your small intestine. After a snack of simple carbohydrates, the pancreas gets a strong, sudden message that a whole lot of sugar has just hit the bloodstream, and it pumps out a lot of insulin to bring blood sugar levels back down. If this happens over and over again, day in and day out, you are setting yourself up for insulin resistance, mood swings, and fatigue. Insulin resistance tends to raise levels of blood fats known as triglycerides, LDL cholesterol, and blood sugar. Chronically increased levels of these substances can lead to obesity, diabetes, heart disease, and a host of other degenerative disorders.

It is wise to read labels carefully and do all you can to avoid foods that contain refined sugars. These can hide out in otherwise nutritious foods. For example, plain yogurt made with live cultures is an excellent source of protein, calcium, and "friendly" bacteria that support digestive health, but low-fat and fruit-added versions usually are loaded with several teaspoons of sugar. Be aware that sugars show up on labels under many different names, including sucrose, maltodextrin, and high-fructose corn syrup. A twelve-ounce can of soda pop has an average of ten to twelve teaspoons of sugar. It is liquid candy!

Incidentally, it is not a good idea to try to avoid sugar by using artificial sweeteners like aspartame (also sold under the brand names Equal and NutraSweet), saccharin (Sweet 'N Low), and the newer acesulfame-K (Sunette, Sweet 'n Safe, Sweet One). Fake sweeteners do not help you to lose weight or kick your sugar habit, and some of them are known to have adverse effects on brain cells. They whet your taste for sugar without satisfying your body's need for nourishment. Aspartame is an *excitotoxin,* which means that it overexcites brain cells to the point where they literally can die. Chronic headaches, seizures, and brain tumors have been linked with aspartame use. Do not expose yourself or your baby to this chemical.

Americans consume a tremendous quantity of artificial sweetener in the form of diet sodas. In addition to containing artificial sweeteners, diet sodas also contain the same load of inorganic phosphorus that regular sodas do, which means that they can throw off your calcium and magnesium balance. We predict that a whole generation of soda-guzzling teens and young adults may well be headed for osteoporosis in their twilight years because of the bone-eroding effects of excess phosphoric acid. The average cola drink is 100,000 times more acidic than the human bloodstream should be, having a a pH of 2 rather than 7. It therefore takes about ten gallons of water to neutralize one can of soda. To bring the blood pH back into balance, the body will rob alkaline minerals from anywhere it can get them, including bone.

Refined Flour

Refined flour—the kind used to make fluffy breads, many breakfast cereals, pretzels, bagels, muffins, cookies, and pasta—is only slightly better for you than sugar. It contains carbohydrates that take a little bit longer to break down than those in pure sugar. Still, it is essentially predigested and causes a big jump in blood sugar. That is why a bagel with jam in the morning only tides you over for an hour or two—your blood sugar soars, then crashes, and you probably find yourself craving more carbohydrates before lunchtime.

If you are trying to lose weight, refined flour products can get you into big trouble because they are highly calorically dense but not very filling. How many times have you polished off several slices of bread in a restaurant before your dinner arrived? By the time you dig in to the main course, you have already had 500 calories' worth of flour—and if you have been slathering butter all over each piece, you are looking at closer to 1,000 calories. The calories your body does not need go right into fat storage, and your blood sugars rise and crash much as they would if you had eaten sugar. Those calories are about as empty as they come.

In addition, many people have allergies to gluten, a protein found in barley, oats, rye, and wheat, and in the wheat alternatives amaranth and spelt. If you find it difficult to have a single meal without something made from wheat, and you have chronic allergies, asthma, or itchy skin rashes, try replacing these foods with products made from brown rice or buckwheat. There are many gluten-free alternatives available in the average health food market. See if you can stay away from gluten-containing foods for at least two weeks. If you do and then see a notable improvement in your allergic symptoms, you may be sensitive to these foods. You should be able to add some gluten-containing foods back to your diet after a while without provoking a reaction, as long as you don't have them every day. Most conventional physicians still rarely acknowledge any but the most extreme cases of food allergy, but we have seen remarkable improvements in people who ferret out and eliminate allergenic foods from their diets. (We will talk more about food allergies in Chapter 8.)

Another problem with a diet rich in refined flour is that it can be incredibly constipating. When you made glue for papier-mâché in grade school, what did you use? Flour and water! The same kind of reaction happens in your gastrointestinal tract when you eat lots of wheat that has been stripped of its oils, its nutritious germ, and its fiber.

Women with gestational diabetes are usually placed on a low- to no-carbohydrate diet, which controls insulin and glucose levels well in most cases. Unless you have been diagnosed with diabetes, you can take a more moderate tack—eating high-fiber foods such as beans, legumes, whole grains, fresh fruits, and vegetables. Protein from lean meats, fresh fish, and poultry can help to quell cravings for sweets and refined flour products. (In many instances, cravings for sugar are a sign that your body needs protein.) Intense cravings for sugar can be a sign that the brain's serotonin levels are too low.

Finally, sugars and refined flour affect the action of enzymes that orchestrate prostaglandin production. If you eat too much of these foods, your body produces more of the "bad" prostaglandins (see page 54).

Kicking the Refined Sugar and Flour Habit

Are you daunted by the notion of kicking your sugar and refined flour habit, although you know that you need to? Not sure how to begin? The best way is to do it cold turkey. On your next shopping expedition, pass by the sweet goodies and the white-flour bread and bagels. Instead, select some whole-grain products, or some whole grains from the bulk section of the market. Fill your cart with fresh vegetables and fruit. For at least three days, commit yourself to eating only whole foods. Steam vegetables, bake yams, eat raw salads, and cook beans and brown rice or rolled oats. Use organic butter, olive oil, tamari (soy sauce), and other savory seasonings, and remember to add some protein to each meal in the form of plain organic yogurt, organic cheeses, nuts, seeds, tofu, fish, or free-range poultry or beef. Don't add concentrated sweeteners to anything. If you want something sweet, eat a piece of fresh fruit. You will find that your taste for the really sweet stuff dissipates quickly. Once you get to this point, you can go back to having an *occasional* sweet or piece of white bread without going overboard.

In general, you can add sweetness to foods with natural sweeteners like maple syrup and honey—but use them judiciously, too. For women who cannot seem to kick their refined carbohydrate cravings, or who choose to be vegetarian or vegan, we prescribe a food supplement powder containing amino acids, vitamins, fiber, and the minerals chromium and vanadium. (More about this in Chapter 7.)

EAT FOODS THAT SUPPLY
YOUR BODY WITH ANTIOXIDANTS

Antioxidants are nutrients that help prevent free radicals from building up in your body and causing damage to the proteins and fats that make up your cells. Free radicals are constantly being formed during the metabolic processes that take place in your mitochondria (see page 37). If your life is in balance and your intake of antioxidants is adequate, you can keep damaging free radicals in check. If you are stressed out, eating poor quality foods, exercising too much or too strenuously, exposed to toxins, or ill, your free-radical burden can build up to levels higher than your antioxidant intake can handle. This is why antioxidant-rich foods are an important part of any diet, especially a diet designed to relieve postpartum complaints and rebuild depleted nutrient stores.

The use of antioxidant supplements in the form of vitamin C, vitamin E, and beta-carotene has become commonplace. This is a good thing, but unless you are taking a very sophisticated antioxidant supplement, these isolated nutrients cannot reproduce the beneficial effects of antioxidants in their naturally occurring forms. When you eat an orange or a peach, there is more to the antioxidants in those fruits than there is to a vitamin-C tablet or a vitamin-E capsule—probably including benefits that we have yet to discover in the field of nutritional science.

If you eat a diet rich in colorful vegetables and fruits, you are getting lots of naturally occurring plant-based antioxidants. Herbs and spices such as rosemary and turmeric are also wonderful sources of antioxidant nutrients. Rosemary contains several different phytochemicals that studies have shown to be antioxidant, anti-inflammatory, and antibacterial. Other research has shown that rosemary supports liver detoxification by boosting levels of antioxidant enzymes known as glutathione-S-transferases and quinone reductases and by inhibiting phase I enzymes that convert chemical toxins to more carcinogenic forms. Turmeric is a spice often used in Indian cooking. It also appears as a natural food coloring in mustard and other foods. The spice itself has long been used in Ayurveda, or traditional Indian medicine. It contains a powerful anti-inflammatory, anti-infective, and antioxidant substance—curcumin—that raises levels of the important antioxidant glutathione in cells throughout the body. It is especially useful for liver diseases such as hepatitis, but everyone—especially those whose detoxification systems have been pushed to their limits by the stresses of pregnancy—can benefit from the beneficial effects of curcumin on glutathione levels. Curcumin can also be used in supplement form to help heal inflammatory conditions and to promote recovery from surgery or strenuous exercise. (Childbirth is about as strenuous as exercise gets.)

EAT SLOWLY AND CHEW YOUR FOOD THOROUGHLY

Eat your meals slowly and deliberately, chewing each bite thoroughly. It is too easy to get into the habit of scarfing down your food when you do not know how long you will be able to sit and eat before being interrupted by your baby. This contributes to digestive troubles and tends to lead to eating more than you really need. If you eat whole foods and chew them completely, you will be amazed at how much better these foods taste—and how quickly you become satiated.

It is important not to let yourself get so famished that you grab whatever edible thing first comes within your reach. If you are going out with your baby, pack some healthy snacks to take along with you. Choose foods that contain a balance of protein, carbohydrate, and fat. Some good ideas include celery or an apple with nut butter, nut and seed trail mix, a cheese or tuna fish sandwich on whole-grain bread with sprouts and tomato, a protein-rich smoothie, or—if you are really pressed—one of the many commercially available protein bars. These bars should be seen as a last resort because they tend to contain refined sugar and other overly refined ingredients, but they are better than a candy bar or a fluffy white-flour pastry.

EAT A SOURCE OF NUTRIENT-LADEN FIBER,
SUCH AS GROUND FLAXSEEDS

While we do not recommend that you ingest significant quantities of flaxseed oil (see page 99), we do recommend that you add whole flaxseeds to your diet in small amounts. Traditionally known as linseeds, flaxseeds are packed with nutrients and fiber, and contain antioxidants that naturally protect against rancidity. They are one of nature's richest sources of ALA, the omega-3 fatty acid, and they contain a type of fiber that is an excellent source of a short-chain fatty acid called *butyrate*. Formed in the colon by the action of friendly bacteria on the flaxseed fiber, butyrate is the fuel preferred over any other by the cells of the large intestine (the colon), and is made when the good bowel flora digests fiber. The colon is not just a tube that carries wastes out of your body. It is actually an entire ecosystem, harboring beneficial bacteria that help your system to better absorb nutrients and get rid of toxins. Maintaining colon health becomes much easier if you eat a whole-foods diet, and by including flaxseeds in that diet you give your colon extra support. (You will learn more about supporting digestive health in Chapter 8.)

Store flaxseeds in a container in your freezer. Grind a small amount (a tablespoon or two) at a time in a coffee grinder and add them to cereals, smoothies, and cooked grains.

A Word about Vegetarian Diets

We appreciate the ethical and moral concerns of those who choose to refrain from the use of animal foods. However, a vegan diet is not the best choice for the pregnant or nursing mother (or, really, the healthiest diet for your body at any point in your life). A nursing or pregnant mother cannot expect to eat a low-fat vegan or vegetarian diet and have a smooth experience during pregnancy and postpartum. Such a diet simply does not give her body the nutrients and healthy fats it needs. Vegan mothers may have an easy time during pregnancy and a positive birth experience, but postpartum ailments are common and subsequent pregnancies tend to be troublesome because of nutrient depletion. Our clinical experience has shown this to us time and time again.

Statistically, vegans do have fewer cases of heart disease than meat-eaters, but we have observed that they seem more vulnerable to colds, flus, structural problems such as joint pain, immune-system problems, and lymphoma. A vegetarian diet that incorporates dairy products and eggs is a step closer to the ideal diet, but it still deprives you of one of the most nourishing foods you can eat, especially during pregnancy and postpartum: deepwater fish.

Many health-conscious vegetarians stop eating meat and dairy products because they want to decrease their fat intake. There is nothing wrong with the fat that nature put into whole foods. When food manufacturers take the fat out, they have to add sugar and flavorings to add back the taste and what food technologists call the "mouth feel" of the full-fat versions. Foods that contain natural fats and proteins are more satisfying, and you need less of them to feel as though you have had enough. Eating meat, dairy products, and eggs does not cause heart disease. The relationship between food and clogged arteries is much more complicated than some people would have us believe. *Moderate* consumption of animal foods, along with lots of vegetables, whole grains, and fruit, will not put you at increased risk for a heart attack.

If you make the choice to stay with a vegan or vegetarian diet because of spiritual or moral concerns, we admire your commitment to your ideals. However, be aware that you need to focus on supplementing the amino acids, healthy fats, and other nutrients that are likely to be lacking in your diet. The information in Chapter 7 will help you to do this.

We realize that if you are not used to eating whole foods and a wide variety of fresh vegetables and whole grains, the lifestyle changes we have suggested in this chapter could seem difficult or daunting. To address those concerns, the next chapter will give you some simple, straightforward suggestions for food preparation.

6

Postpartum Food Preparation: Practical Matters

Once you are through the first couple of weeks postpartum, you will be establishing the rhythm of life with your new baby. If you have not already done so, now is the time for you and your partner to figure out how to fit the preparation of nourishing meals into your lives. You don't need to measure serving sizes, try a lot of exotic new foods, or follow complicated recipes to do this. And you don't have to follow any specific diet "plans" or do any mathematical calculations to figure out how much to eat of certain foods. You have enough to worry about as it is. All you need to do is work within some general guidelines. In the preceding chapter, we looked at guidelines covering which foods to choose. In this chapter, we will look at some practical matters concerning how to use and prepare those foods in the easiest and most healthful way.

Kitchen Basics

Set up your kitchen for the greatest possible ease and convenience. In the past, this may have meant having plenty of frozen pizzas and Lean Cuisine meals and a working microwave, but to make the shift to a whole-foods diet, you need a few other gadgets, including the following:

- A blender.
- A small coffee bean or seed grinder.
- A food processor.
- A rice cooker.
- A salad spinner.
- A slow cooker (Crock-Pot).
- Freezer bags, small and large varieties.
- Glass canning jars (Mason jars).
- Reusable plastic storage containers (Tupperware or similar brands).

Having all of these items on hand will help you to simplify the processes of cooking and storing healthful food with a minimum of work time in the kitchen.

At the Grocery Store

First, if at all possible, find a grocery in your area that sells organic produce, meats, and dairy products. Be prepared to spend a bit more than you are used to on these staples. Remind yourself that your family's health is worth the extra money. If you have a local farmers' market, shop there for produce. Your baby will love the sights, sounds, and scents of the farmers' market, and later will enjoy the taste of the produce.

If your experience with vegetables has been limited to overcooked broccoli smothered with cheddar cheese sauce and iceberg lettuce salad, you have a whole wonderful new world of tastes waiting for you. When you walk into the market, however, you may find yourself more intimidated than excited. Here is a starter list of vegetables to try. You should have enough vegetables in the house to provide some for each meal. It will take a few weeks of trial and error to figure out how much you need and which varieties taste best to you.

- Artichoke.
- Asparagus.
- Beans (French or green).
- Beets.
- Broccoli.
- Brussels sprouts.
- Butternut or other type of winter squash.
- Cabbage.
- Carrots.
- Cauliflower.
- Celery.
- Chard or kale.
- Corn.
- Eggplant.
- Jicama.
- Leeks.
- Lima beans.
- Mushrooms.
- Onions.
- Peas.
- Potatoes.
- Spinach.
- Sprouts (try alfalfa, broccoli, garbanzo, lentil, mung bean, and other sprouted nuts, beans, and seeds).
- Sweet bell peppers (red, yellow, orange, or green).
- Sweet potatoes or garnet yams.
- Tomatoes.
- Turnips.
- Yellow squash.
- Zucchini.

In addition to fresh vegetables, keep some frozen ones on hand in case you run out of everything else. Frozen spinach is especially handy in a pinch—it can be scrambled into eggs, stirred into a marinara sauce, or steamed and eaten on its own. Many natural food stores now carry frozen organic vegetables.

Choose fruits in season, preferably ones grown near where you live. Apples are one of our favorites. Organic purple grapes, cherries, blueberries, and mangoes are packed with antioxidant nutrients. Organic melons, peaches, and plums are also winners. Many health food markets carry organic bananas. Try some unsweetened organic applesauce for a snack or dessert. Avocado is rich in healthy fats and is great when mashed to make a spread or vegetable dip. Or stuff half an avocado with tuna, celery, and scallions mixed with a little canola mayonnaise for a quick, satisfying meal. (Mashed avocado is also an ideal early food for baby!) Also buy canned beans: black beans, garbanzo beans, kidney beans, and/or white beans. These can be added to rice for a quick meal, or to soups for protein.

Shop for cold-water fish such as salmon, cod, and mackerel. Buy canned sardines or anchovies to keep in the pantry. Canned tuna is all right once weekly, but mercury naturally accumulates in its flesh so it should not be eaten excessively. Plan to eat fish two to three times weekly.

If you like nut butters, try raw almond butter, cashew butter, or sesame butter. We do not recommend peanut butter for nursing mothers. Some data suggest that babies can develop an allergy to peanuts if the mother eats them while breastfeeding.

If you love fruit juice but do not have a juicer at home, buy natural fruit juices without added sugar, flavorings, or corn syrup. If you are nursing, avoid citrus juices. Try papaya, apple, or grape juice instead.

Most health food markets now sell several varieties of boxed broth such as organic chicken, vegetable, and mushroom. Keep a few boxes in your pantry and use for quick soups or for cooking more flavorful whole grains. Check the labels to make sure they contain only ingredients you recognize—and that they don't contain monosodium glutamate (MSG), which is often disguised as hydrolyzed vegetable protein.

If you enjoy bread, go for those made from whole, sprouted grains, such as Ezekiel bread (also sometimes called Bible bread or fasting bread). This type of bread rarely contains preservatives, so keep it in the freezer. Manna bread is a good, dense whole-grain bread. Some artisan bakeries still make traditional breads from rye, sourdough, and whole wheat flour. If you are lucky enough to have one of these bakeries in your town, you can indulge in their breads once in a while. You can also try mochi, a chewy rice bread that you bake in the oven and cut into squares—look in the refrigerated section of your health food market. Corn tortillas or whole-wheat chapatis, a type of Indian bread, are good bread alternatives. If you are sensitive to gluten, you can try gluten-free breads made from rice flour and nuts. You should be able to find these in your health food market. Toast them for better texture and flavor.

Stock up on brown rice, quinoa (pronounced *KEEN-wah*), and barley in the bulk section. If you are feeling adventurous, try amaranth, millet, or kasha (roasted buckwheat).

Keep a container of miso in your refrigerator. This can be used to add flavor to soups and stews, and it makes a great broth—simply boil water, turn off the heat, stir in miso, and add chopped scallions, strips of kombu seaweed (which is great in other soups, too—find it at an Asian grocery or in your health food market), and small cubes of tofu.

If you don't already have them, purchase a variety of spices and herbs. Some of the basics are basil, cayenne pepper, curry powder, dill, dry mustard, garlic powder, herbs de Provence (a mixture of several herbs that is delicious in omelets, on fish, and in soups), rosemary, sage, and thyme. Chopped or minced fresh garlic that comes in a jar is a valuable time-saver, as are chopped basil and pesto (a mixture of basil, garlic, olive oil, and pine nuts). When you shop for any type of condiment (or any processed foods), check the label first to make sure it does not contain dyes, flavor enhancers such as MSG, or artificial preservatives. Keep prepared salsas and organic sauces, marinades, and condiments in your kitchen to quickly add zing to meat and egg dishes.

Get yourself a supply of a few different salad dressings—a vinaigrette, a creamy ranch, caesar, or bleu cheese dressing, and a tahini-based dressing (but make sure to choose brands that are *not* made with hydrogenated oils). At the dairy case, choose one or two varieties of organic cheese if you like to eat cheeses. Feta and aged cheddar are so flavorful that you don't need to use much to spice things up.

Other staples to purchase include organic butter or ghee (clarified butter), organic plain yogurt, maple syrup, honey, and rice milk.

Tips for Speeding Food Preparation

Two or three times a week, take an hour's time to prepare foods for easy cooking. Hand baby over to Dad and cook, chop, dice, and store some basics (or have Dad handle the kitchen chores):

- Hard-boil a half-dozen eggs, peel off the shells, and store them in a plastic container.
- Wash and cut up raw vegetables such as beets, bell peppers, carrots, celery, cucumber, jicama, and radishes, and store them in plastic containers in the refrigerator. These are great for snacks or for quick salad preparation.
- Wash and remove the ribs and stems from chard, collards, kale, spinach, and/or other greens. Keep these in airtight plastic bags in the fridge. Then, when you want to add cooked greens to a meal, you can pour them right into your stir-fry pan with a few tablespoons of water, a dash of olive oil, some tamari, and as much garlic as you like, and allow the greens to cook until soft.
- Cut up leeks, onions, scallions, yellow squash, and/or zucchini and store the pieces in plastic containers for steaming, stir-frying, or use in soups. You can freeze most vegetables.
- If you like winter squash, cut them in half, scoop out any seeds, and roast face up in a baking pan filled a half-inch up with water, in a 425°F oven for about an hour. You can chop up apples or nuts to put in the middle. Then you can either scoop the flesh out of the skin and eat it right away, store the cooked squash in an airtight plastic container to eat later, or blend it with vegetable or chicken broth to make soup.
- Keep your salad spinner filled with washed baby greens, Boston (Bibb) lettuce, or romaine.

- Cook asparagus, broccoli, cauliflower, and/or garnet yams ahead of time and keep them in the refrigerator for a cold meal or snack. (You may not be able to imagine eating baked yams without marshmallows—but try them split open hot with a pat of butter or some olive oil, some prepared garlic right out of the jar, and a dash of soy sauce inside.) Chilled steamed vegetables are great in salads.
- Divide fresh fish into 3-ounce portions—about the size of a deck of cards. Freeze individual portions wrapped in wax paper and sealed in airtight plastic bags. (Fish must be frozen in sealed airtight containers or it will go bad.) You can later move them into the refrigerator on the morning of the day you plan to have fish for dinner, or quick-thaw an individual portion in a bowl of warm water for an hour before you cook it. Freeze boneless chicken breasts in individual portions as well, or roast a whole free-range chicken and keep in the refrigerator. You can pull some meat from it to add to salads or soups, or to make a sandwich.
- Keep whole grains in glass canning jars with easy-to-read labels. Also keep nuts and seeds in clearly labeled glass jars. Toasted pumpkinseeds or walnuts are especially good additions to salad, and both are rich sources of alpha-linolenic acid (ALA). You can toast them in a dry skillet over low heat, stirring often until you can smell the toastiness or the seeds begin to pop. Or spread them on a baking sheet and toast them in a preheated 250°F oven for about ten minutes.

With these basic preparations done, cooking meals will be easier and quicker.

Menu Planning

If you are not familiar with preparing vegetables and whole grains, invest in a few vegetarian or whole-foods cookbooks to learn how to simply prepare vegetables and whole grains. Cooking whole grains in a rice cooker is as easy as adding one part grain to two parts liquid (water or broth) and turning it on. The cooker will turn itself off when the grain is cooked. Add flavor with a dash of tamari (soy sauce) and a small pat of organic butter or ghee. Use uncooked grains when making soup, or add leftover cooked grains after the soup is cooked.

Add small amounts of meat or fish to vegetarian fare for flavorful, well-rounded meals. Recommended types of meat include free-range beef, lamb, and poultry, or game meats such as venison or buffalo. Think of meats as side dishes and veggies and grains as your main courses. If you eat according to our guidelines, your protein intake will be balanced and adequate, and you will not need to make any special adjustments to ensure that you are getting enough protein. Even if you prefer to refrain from meat other than fish, your two-to-three-times-weekly fish and omega-3 eggs on other days of the week will satisfy your protein requirements.

Many nursing mothers find that they crave meat more than they did before they were pregnant. You can follow this craving as long as you avoid fast-food burgers and fried meats. Always eat a substantial amount of vegetables with meat to help keep the acid/alkaline ratio balanced in your body.

Don't feel you need to adhere to recipes exactly—just use them to get a feel for which herbs and spices go best with which whole foods and for basic cooking guidelines. *The Co-Op Cookbook: Delicious and Healthy Meals in Less Than Half an Hour* by Rosemary Fifield (Chelsea Green Publishing Company, 2000) is a great cookbook that contains lots of simple, fast, wholesome recipes. *Feeding the Whole Family: Whole Foods Recipes for Babies, Young Children and Their Parents* by Cynthia Lair (Moon Smile Publishers, 1998) is another great resource that can help you to incorporate natural whole foods into your childrens' diets from the time they are ready to eat solid foods. Other good cookbooks include *Nourishing Traditions* by Sally Fallon (New Trends Publishing, 1999); any of the Moosewood series by Mollie Katzen and the Moosewood Collective (these have had a number of different publishers over the years); and *A Vegetarian's Ecstasy* by Natalie Cederquist and James Levin (Avery Publishing Group, 1996).

Soups and salads are the quickest and easiest ways to get good nutrition without spending a lot of time at food preparation. You can make soups or stews in a slow cooker, so that you can have a hot meal without putting in much time in the kitchen. Soups with well-cooked fish, meat, poultry, legumes, whole grains, and vegetables are easy to digest and contain the nutrients you and your baby need. Just fill a pot with prepared broth and add chopped vegetables, meat, beans, and a grain, and simmer until the grain is cooked.

If you plan to have a soup or stew once a day, a salad once a day, and a protein-and-grain meal once a day, you have covered all of your bases!

Let us look at an example of how all this might come together in a day's meals.

BREAKFAST

A good breakfast could consist of one or two hard-boiled DHA eggs with sprouted grain toast, or three-grain cereal composed of one part quinoa, one part millet, and one part amaranth, cooked in your rice cooker. Before eating the cereal, you can stir in pure maple syrup or honey and rice milk, or add fresh fruit or a dollop of plain yogurt. You can eat any leftover grains with veggies and chicken for lunch or dinner.

Don't rule out having soup for breakfast. A steaming bowl of vegetable-beef, chicken, or fish soup with a warm chunk of whole-grain bread topped with butter or melted cheese is much more satisfying and nutritious than a bowl of sweetened cereal!

Smoothies make a great hot-weather breakfast or snack. Grind 1 tablespoon of raw flaxseeds in a blender or coffee grinder. Add the resulting flaxseed meal to 2 cups of apple, pear, or papaya juice, or to two cups of rice milk; then add one banana and ¼ to ½ cup of frozen blueberries or strawberries. Blend until smooth. Try other fruits or juices, too. You can add spirulina powder for extra B vitamins and antioxidant vitamins. You can also add some protein powder for extra amino acids.

SNACKS

When you need a snack to keep your energy up, choose a healthful, nutrient-rich one such as the following:

- Organic applesauce.
- A smoothie (see the previous section on breakfast).
- Fresh fruit or vegetables with protein—for example, a sliced apple spread with almond butter, or celery sticks spread with cashew butter, or carrot sticks dipped in tahini dressing.
- Nuts.
- A slice of whole-grain bread with nut butter, organic cheese, tuna, or sardines.

LUNCH AND DINNER

Salads make excellent and easy meals or components of meals. Simply mix and match the ingredients kept in your refrigerator. Start with torn pieces of lettuce or spring greens and add grated beets and/or carrots, bean sprouts, chilled steamed asparagus or broccoli, and a protein source such as grilled fish or chicken. Slices of avocado are a tasty addition, rich in healthy fats. Top with toasted pumpkin or sunflower seeds if you like.

For a grain/vegetable/protein meal, try salmon with brown rice and chard or chicken with quinoa and green beans. You can also leave out the grain and have two vegetables; try turkey with garnet yams and sweet peas, or lamb with zucchini and new potatoes. Another tasty option: black beans, chicken, or cod; avocado slices; and thinly sliced raw cabbage (if it agrees with your baby) with salsa, served with warm corn tortillas. Add grated cheese if you like.

Soups are always good choices. Cut up some onion, carrot, and celery, and place them in your slow cooker. Add ½ cup lentils, 4 cups of mushroom or vegetable broth, a pound of lamb for stewing, and torn pieces of kale and/or chard. Add four diced tomatoes and a handful of diced red or green bell pepper, add water if necessary for consistency, and let the soup simmer for four hours. You can walk away from your Crock-Pot and go about your day while your soup cooks. Season the soup with whatever herbs you like. (Most canned broths contain salt, so you shouldn't need to add more.)

Alternatively, try four cans or two boxes of organic chicken broth and add various chopped vegetables—such as onion, celery, carrot, zucchini, yellow squash, peppers, green beans, peas, potato, and spinach. Add ¼ to ½ cup barley and diced chicken thighs or breast and allow the mixture to simmer for four hours in a slow cooker.

Making a creamy soup is easy with prepared broth. Bake a butternut squash and put the baked flesh into a blender with 4 cups of broth and blend until smooth. You can sip this soup hot or cold.

Getting the Hang of the Postpartum Diet Plan

When it comes to establishing healthy new ways of eating, pay attention to what works best for your body. Some people enjoy tofu, while others find that this soy product gives them indigestion. Some do well with dairy products, while others end up with runny noses or diarrhea when they eat dairy foods. Keep in mind that calcium is present in virtually all vegetables and nuts, so if you eat plenty of those, you don't need to drink milk to get enough calcium in your diet, even though you are using a lot of your calcium stores to make milk for your baby.

Remember that you are unique, and the postpartum diet that works for you will be unique, too. Work within the guidelines in this chapter according to your own tastes and your own instincts about what foods make you feel the most energetic and clearheaded. All it requires is that you pay attention to how your body responds to the foods you eat. When so much of your energy is focused on caring for an infant, it can be hard to do this, but once you have established your ideal postpartum diet, you will feel it hasn't been a wasted effort. If you are lucky enough to be reading this book before or during pregnancy, you can start changing the way you eat now.

Of course, you will have "lapses" from your new healthy diet. One day, you might really want that fast-food burger; another day you might be satisfied only by a big candy bar or ice-cream sundae. Go ahead and allow yourself the occasional indulgence. Perfection is not something that humans should expect of themselves! In fact, if you allow yourself the occasional indulgence, you are far more likely to avoid bingeing. Just don't use a temporary indulgence as a reason to feel bad and slide back into a day-to-day way of eating that won't nourish your body or your baby's body.

7

Building Nutrient Reserves
with Supplements

Should you be able to get all the nutrition you need from a good diet? This is the million-dollar question, debated by medical and nutrition experts worldwide. If you have a sizeable organic garden in your yard, and you harvest vegetables and fruit from that garden year-round and eat them the day they are harvested, and you live a relatively balanced, stress-free life, get enough exercise and sleep, and are not chronically exposed to pollutants, and you have perfect health and digestion, then yes—you can *probably* get all the vitamins, minerals, and accessory nutrients you require from the foods you eat. If you are an urban or suburban dweller who hunts and gathers at the grocery store, eats fast food from time to time, and lives a typically new-millennium fast-paced life, we strongly recommend that you consider using nutritional supplements to rebuild and maintain your nutrient reserves. This recommendation is based upon looking at thousands of sophisticated blood tests that measure many types of nutrient deficiencies. Everyone tested had deficiencies in at least a few nutrients essential to good health. Recent studies reveal that because the soil in the United States has lost almost half of its original mineral content due to farming methods that do not focus on soil nutrient replenishment, most foods bought in the grocery store have only a fraction of the nutrient content they contained a few decades ago. This dramatically reduces your chances of getting all the nutrients your body needs from food sources alone. Let us review some of the reasons why supplements can be so important for maintaining optimal health.

Conventionally grown vegetables and fruits are rarely given the opportunity to ripen on the plant from which they grew. The antioxidant vitamins and accessory nutrients—natural plant chemicals that are not categorized as vitamins or minerals but that have supportive and healing effects on the body—in those foods that develop fully during the natural ripening process, are never allowed to come forth. Instead, fruits and vegetables are picked unripe and often end up being shipped halfway across the continent—if not halfway around the world—before they arrive at your grocery store. Every day that a piece of fruit or a vegetable is off of the plant, it loses nutrients. The lack of nutrients in these foods is what makes them bland and colorless when compared with the locally grown, organic produce you might see at a farmers' market or health food store.

Compare a typical supermarket tomato with an organically grown one. The supermarket tomato might be blemish-free and large, but it contains far fewer nutrients than the more deeply hued organic variety. If you taste a slice of each, you will realize that there is no contest when it comes to flavor, consistency, and aroma. You can drop the average conventionally farmed tomato to the ground from four feet up without breaking it open, while the more delicate organic tomato may have the occasional bruise, blemish, or bug. Tomatoes grown organically and locally are sweet, tender, and succulent, while conventional tomatoes tend to be tasteless, tough, or mealy.

The genetic engineering of plants has allowed us to breed produce that looks nice, despite its having been shipped across several states, or even across oceans. This kind of engineering of plants makes things easier on the grocer, but the consumer ends up with food that does not supply adequate nutrition.

Conventionally farmed produce also contains far more *antinutrients* than organically farmed produce. Chemical pesticides and herbicides that are sprayed on conventional produce are major sources of antinutrients. As discussed in Chapter 3, the nutrients stored up in your tissues are used in the detoxification processes that rid your body of toxins such as synthetic chemicals. In other words, antinutrient-laden foods actually *increase* your body's demand for vitamins and minerals, even as they fail to fulfill your body's need for those nutrients.

We know that many pesticides contain chemicals called *xenohormones,* a term that refers to hormones that come from the environment. Xenohormones can mimic the effects of natural hormones in the body in a way that threatens the integrity of the genetic material that keeps cells healthy. The testing for the safety of these chemicals is woefully inadequate. Because they are only tested individually, we really have no idea how these chemicals interact in the body.

Cattle, pigs, and poultry raised on factory farms eat antinutrient-loaded feed and those antinutrients become concentrated in their meat, eggs, and milk. The further up the food chain antinutrients go, the more concentrated they become. Mother's milk is at the highest rung on the food chain, providing an even more concentrated source of these chemicals that passes into your baby's body. This is why it is so important to try to eat organic foods as much as possible while you are pregnant and nursing.

Unfortunately, some exposure to antinutrients is unavoidable; humankind has done a tremendous job of making its toxic mark from sea to shining sea, to the depths of the deepest oceans, and to the farthest reaches of the Arctic. Thus, you should do all you can to avoid antinutrients by eating organic foods whenever possible, but you should also fortify your body's defenses by giving your body the nutrients it needs to effectively detoxify antinutrients. Along with a whole-foods, mostly organic diet, smart nutritional supplementation will do just that.

A Scientific Approach to Nutrient Supplementation

If you feel overwhelmed by the hype that has surrounded the use of supplements, you are not alone. A huge, largely unregulated industry has been created to supply the public with supplemental nutrients. There is certainly no shortage of information about nutritional products in print and online, but not all of it is backed by sound clinical research. It can feel like a leap of faith to choose from the huge number of available nutritional products. Try to find products that have passed the rigors of U.S. Food and Drug Administration (FDA) approved clinical research studies to ensure effectiveness and safety.

Functional medicine takes a scientific approach to nutrient supplementation. We live in a scientific age, and sound science is the best way to show the value of a nutritional product. This is so even with herbs and medicinal foods, which have been used for millennia to heal all manner of ills without so much as a laboratory assay. Just as we can see what is lacking at the cellular level with laboratory testing, we also have the capability to observe how nutrients work to support health at the cellular level. Functional medicine uses that capability to obtain a clear view of what really works—which takes the guesswork out of it for you. A scientific approach also allows us to discover which forms of various nutrients are best absorbed and utilized by the body.

The balance of this chapter will give you some general guidelines for a nutrient supplementation program. You will find out what these nutrients do in your body and what problems they can help to relieve. These guidelines can be used by every woman who reads this book, although, depending on the results of your lab tests, you may need to add other nutrients or use more of the ones listed here. As you read along, you will gain insight into how you might individualize your supplement program according to your own deficiencies and symptoms. We do recommend, especially if you have any kind of serious illness, that you choose a qualified health practitioner who can run laboratory tests for you at regular intervals. Nutritional testing, initially done every three to six months, helps your practitioner to determine how well your body is absorbing the nutrients that have been prescribed and when and how to adjust dosages. If your lab results indicate a more serious disease process, your health practitioner may choose to treat this or refer you to an appropriate medical specialist.

Prenatal and Postpartum Multivitamin and Mineral Supplements

We recommend that you make a high-quality multivitamin and mineral supplement a part of your daily routine for the rest of your life. The consistent use of a multivitamin and mineral supplement does not make up for a poor diet, but it will help to ensure that your basic nutrient needs are covered. We feel that doctors who tell their patients that they can get all the nutrients they need from a "well-balanced diet" are not being realistic. Precious few of the doctors that make this kind of statement have any experience with the type of nutritional testing discussed in this book. There are too many internal and external nutrient-depleting factors working against us to rely solely on food for all the nutrients we need to be truly healthy. It is very difficult to replenish significantly depleted nutrient reserves by food alone. The use of nutraceuticals—nutrients concentrated to higher, therapeutic dosages—is the most effective way we have found to replenish your body's reserves of depleted nutrients.

Nutrient requirements vary widely. One woman might not need much more than a multivitamin/mineral supplement to get back on her feet after pregnancy, while another might need to take several other supplements in addition to her multivitamin/mineral to bring her body back into balance. Some of this variability depends on what you eat, the efficiency of your digestive tract, and the amount of stress you are under; some will hinge on your individual genetic makeup.

What constitutes a "high-quality" multivitamin and mineral supplement? Look for one that contains the forms of the vitamins and minerals that are best assimilated (absorbed and used by the body). Expect to take three to nine tablets a day, in divided doses—two or three with each meal. If you have trouble swallowing pills, look for a powdered form that can be stirred into juice or blended into a smoothie.

Our recommendations are the average daily doses to look for. This does not mean you should go above that dosage for general health and well-being. With vitamins and minerals, more is not better unless you have specific needs validated by lab tests. Choose a multivitamin and mineral supplement that offers something close to these recommendations. Later we will tell you about nutritional testing that can reveal which specific nutrients may be needed to fulfill the individual needs of your own unique body. If your multivitamin and mineral supplement falls short of these minimum recommendations, add more of specific nutrients as needed. (See Table 7.1 on page 137 for a quick reference list of nutrients a basic multivitamin and mineral supplement should contain, and what the recommended daily dose for each nutrient is.)

VITAMIN A

Vitamin A participates in your body's visual, immune, and reproductive functions. It is also needed for the detoxification of harmful chemicals such as dioxin and polychlorinated biphenyls (PCBs).

Egg yolks, whole milk, and liver are the most abundant food sources of preformed vitamin A. (*Preformed* simply means vitamin A that it is not made by the body from carotenoids, but exists in the form of vitamin A in the food or supplement.) Cod liver oil contains vitamin A as well. If you are generally healthy, you do not actually need to have much more than 1,000 to 2,500 international units of vitamin A in your multivitamin supplement; as long as it contains the recommended amount of carotenoids, you can get enough preformed A from your DHA eggs.

If your eyes, skin, and the mucous membranes in your nose or mouth tend to be dry and rough, you may be deficient in vitamin A. Adding carotenoids (see below) may help, but it is possible that you will need some preformed A to replenish your nutrient stores. If you are catching every flu and cold that comes your way, get frequent sore throats, or are having repeated breast infections or other infections, you may benefit from 1,000 to 5,000 international units of supplemental preformed vitamin A daily. Be aware that high doses of vitamin A (greater than 5,000 international units) should *not* be used during pregnancy because there is an associated risk of birth defects. If you are pregnant and cannot find a doctor to assess your vitamin A levels by means of a blood test, we recommend that you choose a prenatal multivitamin with *no* preformed vitamin A included. For postpartum women, 1,000 to 5,000 international units of vitamin A is usually sufficient, unless a blood test reveals a significant deficiency. A serum concentration below 20 micromoles of vitamin A per deciliter (µg/dL) of blood indicates a long-standing low tissue reserve of this vitamin.

CAROTENOIDS

The carotenoids are a rather large family of plant chemicals that have potent antioxidant activity. They support the body in its efforts to rid itself of toxins and protect itself against the buildup of free radicals. Many of the carotenes can be transformed into vitamin A in the body. This transformation happens more efficiently in some people than in others. You should be getting 1,000 to 10,000 international units of beta-carotene, the best known of these compounds, along with another 1,000 to 10,000 units of mixed carotenoids, daily.

THE B VITAMINS

This group of vitamins, known as the B complex, works as a team to support mitochondrial energy production and nervous system function. For the treatment of specific health problems, you can take higher doses of individual B vitamins. A daily multivitamin should contain the whole B complex in balanced amounts, including 10 to 100 milligrams of vitamin B_1 (thiamin), 5 to 50 milligrams of vitamin B_2 (riboflavin), 25 to 100 milligrams of vitamin B_3 (niacin), 50 to 100 milligrams of pantothenic acid (sometimes referred to to as vitamin B_5), 50 to 100 milligrams of vitamin B_6 (pyridoxine), 100 to 500 micrograms of vitamin B_{12} (cyanocobalamin), 100 to 500 micrograms of biotin, and 400 to 800 micrograms of folic acid.

If you suffer from depression, dry and scaly skin, fatigue, or headaches, you may require higher doses (up to 200 milligrams) of vitamins B_1, B_2, B_3, or B_6; biotin, and/or pantothenic acid. In that case, try taking a B-complex supplement in addition to your multivitamin.

The active form of vitamin B_6, pyridoxyl-5-phosphate (P5P), has helped many women seeking relief from pregnancy-related nausea and is essential for the conversion of the amino acid compound 5-hydroxytryptophan (5-HTP) into the neurotransmitter serotonin. If you can find a multiple vitamin that contains this more expensive form of vitamin B_6, we believe that the benefits will be worth the slight extra expense.

Therapeutic doses of vitamin B_{12} have been used to treat anemia, asthma, depression, and fatigue. If you suffer from severe fatigue during or after pregnancy, try taking up to 5,000 micrograms of extra B_{12} a day. This is a safe way to energize your body and it will not harm your baby. Because there are no good vegetarian food sources of this vitamin, those who want to stick to a vegetarian diet should be sure to supplement with vitamin B_{12}. (Vegetarian forms of B_{12} supplements are available—ask your health-care provider or health food store personnel.) A sublingual supplement (a form designed to be dissolved under the tongue) is best. Vitamin B_{12} needs just the right environment in the digestive system to be absorbed efficiently. Sublingual supplements pass directly into the tiny blood vessels beneath the tongue and into your system. It is not unusual for people who are consuming perfectly adequate amounts of vitamin B_{12} to be deficient because they are not absorbing enough. Supplements that support digestive health (a subject that we discuss later in this chapter) will help create this environment.

Folic acid, also known as folate, is known to prevent neural tube defects—the class of abnormalities that includes spina bifida—in a developing fetus. The most crucial time to get adequate folate is before conception and during the first weeks of pregnancy. Folic acid also works with vitamins B_6 and B_{12} to lower levels of the harmful amino acid homocysteine in the body. These vitamins are required for the metabolism of the amino acid methionine to another amino acid, called cysteine. If not enough of these vitamins is present, homocysteine—an intermediate product of methionine metabolism—builds up in the body. Homocysteine is damaging to the insides of blood vessels. It is a known factor in cardiovascular disease and and may also contribute to Alzheimer's disease, cancer, and nervous-system damage. Thus, ensuring an adequate B-vitamin intake is important not only for a healthy pregnancy, a healthy baby, and immediate postpartum recovery—it will also help to ensure that you will be around to greet your grandchildren when they come into the world! If lab tests show that you have high levels of homocysteine, you can lower them by taking vitamins B_6, B_{12}, folic acid, and another nutrient, betaine. If this is not effective, you may need to use a vitamin formula that contains P5P, a form of folate called 5-methyltetrahydrofolate, or a substance called *intrinsic factor,* which is produced in the stomach and aids in the absorption of vitamin B$_{12}$.

During illness or periods of high stress, the body uses up the B-complex vitamins more quickly, so you may want to consider having an extra B-complex on hand.

VITAMIN C

Your body needs vitamin C to build connective tissues. It is an essential ingredient of collagen, a type of protein that is the raw material from which skin, mucous membranes, gums, and other tissues are made. Vitamin C also activates the immune system, revving up the activity of immune cells that target, destroy, and engulf disease-causing invaders. It works along with vitamins A and E to protect your body against the buildup of free radicals and is needed to make many of the body's hormones. The multivitamin and mineral supplement you choose should provide a minimum of 250 to 1,000 milligrams of vitamin C daily.

During times of stress, your body uses significantly more vitamin C than it does at other times. This vitamin is used to build hormones called *catecholamines* (cat-uh-KOHL-uh-meens), which are produced more rapidly during stressful periods. If you are stressed out or coming down with a virus or bacterial infection, do not hesitate to add an extra few thousand milligrams of vitamin C to your supplement regimen. Doses more than ten times higher than our minimum recommendation have been used without any harm other than a temporary case of diarrhea. Nursing mothers can take up to 1,000 milligrams every couple of hours as soon as they feel a cold or flu taking hold, and baby will get some extra C through mother's milk to protect him against infection.

BIOFLAVONOIDS

Bioflavonoids are a class of phytochemicals that contribute to the bright, beautiful colors of plants. They are powerful antioxidants that work

alongside vitamins and whole-food antioxidants—vitamin C in particular—to protect against free-radical damage. They help to maintain balanced immune function, revving up disease-fighting cells while toning
down the harmful effects of the inflammation that can result when your
body is mounting its defenses against disease. If your multivitamin does
not contain mixed citrus bioflavonoids, consider adding 100 to 250 milligrams a day to your supplement plan.

Proanthocyanidins

Proanthocyanidins (PCOs) give deep purple, blue, and green fruits and vegetables their hue. PCOs are found abundantly in cranberries, blueberries,
and grapes. Have you ever used cranberry extract or cranberry juice to fight
off a urinary tract infection? It is now thought that it is the PCOs in the fruit
and juice that do the work of preventing bacteria from adhering to the
lining of the urinary tract. Grapeseed extract and pine bark extract (sold
under the trademarked name Pycnogenol) are commonly used to make
PCO supplements, but blueberries and cranberries are also rich sources.

PCOs can be considered the "Cadillac of bioflavonoids." They are
more expensive than other bioflavonoids, but they are also more potent.
If you are generally healthy, you will probably do fine with mixed bioflavonoids or quercetin, which are less expensive. If you have a very weak
immune system or are under severe physical or emotional stress, you may
want to invest in PCO supplements for a while. PCOs are also useful for
circulatory problems such as varicose veins—a common complaint during
and after pregnancy. An appropriate dose of PCOs will fall between 150
and 300 milligrams a day.

Quercetin

Quercetin is a bioflavonoid found in the skins of apples and onions. It can
help suppress flareups of viral infections such as herpes. It also dampens
the over-the-top immune system response typical of allergic people. When
a susceptible individual is exposed to an allergen, certain immune cells,
called *mast cells,* release a chemical called *histamine.* In the right amounts,
histamine is not a "bad guy"—in fact, it is vital for effective immunity—
but in those who are allergic, it is a matter of having too much of a good

thing. Runny nose, itchy and watery eyes, and constricted lungs result as histamine works to rid the body of whatever substance has caused the reaction. Therapeutic doses of quercetin can calm histamine release. For allergies, asthma, and hay fever, try taking 500 to 1,500 milligrams of quercetin per day, in divided doses.

Rutin

Rutin is a bioflavonoid that is very important for helping to keep blood vessels strong. Your multivitamin and mineral supplement should provide 20 to 100 milligrams of rutin daily.

VITAMIN D

This "vitamin" is actually a hormonelike biochemical that your body can manufacture when your skin is exposed to sunlight. It regulates the absorption of calcium in the small intestines and the deposition of calcium into bone cells, as well as regulating overall calcium balance throughout the body. Before vitamin D was routinely added to dairy foods, the vitamin D deficiency diseases rickets (in children) and osteomalacia (in adults)—both of which render the bones abnormally soft and weak— were much more common than they are today.

During the first six months of life, your baby requires 300 international units of vitamin D daily. From six months until age ten, she needs 400 international units a day of vitamin D. The multivitamin and mineral supplement you take should give you 400 international units each day. As long as you are getting that amount, along with some sun exposure, you will have enough for both yourself and your baby. Only ten minutes of exposure to summer sunshine stimulates the production of 400 international units of vitamin D in your skin. If you live in an area where sunshine is a rarity, supplemental vitamin D is an especially good idea. Because vitamin D can accumulate in the body, do not take higher than recommended doses except under the supervision of a qualified health-care professional.

VITAMIN E

Vitamin E is an antioxidant vitamin that prevents free radicals from forming in the polyunsaturated fats (PUFAs) that make up cell membranes. Omega-3 and omega-6 fats are PUFAs and are easily oxidized, or harmed by free radicals. These fats make up most of the fats in the membranes that surround each cell in the body. Cells in the nervous system, lungs, and immune system have an especially high need for vitamin E. This vitamin is also needed for optimal immune system function.

Free radicals are molecules or portions of molecules that are chemically unstable because they contain at least one unpaired electron (in stable molecules, all of the electrons occur in pairs). When an antioxidant "quenches" a free radical, it does so by donating an electron to that free radical. This leaves the antioxidant without an electron, which means it itself is then in an unbalanced state and can begin to act like a free radical itself. You might liken this situation to a schoolyard fight over a toy: If Jimmy snatches a toy from Tommy, Jimmy may be less likely to snatch toys from other children, but now Tommy has no toy to play with and might begin to snatch toys from others—unless another child is willing to give a toy to him. Antioxidants can be likened to that generous child.

The are two major forms of vitamin E. The most common forms are called *tocopherols* by nutritionists. The other forms are called *tocotrienols*. Foods contain an array of tocopherols that work cooperatively in your body. Choose a vitamin-E supplement made with mixed tocopherols, including gamma-tocopherol. Avoid products that use the synthetic forms of vitamin E. These are usually denoted by the use of the letters *dl-* at the beginning of the name. For instance, d-alpha-tocopherol is a natural source of vitamin E, while dl-alpha-tocopherol is synthetic. The recommended daily dose of vitamin E in a multivitamin formula is 100 to 400 international units. Tocotrienols are usually not included in any significant amount in multivitamin formulas because they are expensive. High dosages of mixed tocotrienols (200 to 400 international units daily) can be helpful for lowering elevated levels of oxidized low-density lipoprotein (LDL, or "bad") cholesterol.

VITAMIN K

Vitamin K's roles in your body include the maintenance of normal blood clotting and the formation of new bone cells. Newborns in hospitals are routinely given vitamin K shots soon after being born to stave off any possibility of hemorrhage. It is possible that vitamin K therapy could help women with menorrhagia, or extremely heavy menstrual periods.

Outright deficiency of vitamin K used to be rare, because it is made by the friendly bacteria that live in the large intestine. These days, with the broad scope use of antibiotics, which kill off the friendly bowel bacteria that make vitamin K along with the bacteria that cause illness, vitamin K deficiency is becoming much more common than it used to be. For this reason, we feel it is wise to have a supplement that gives you 50 to 100 micrograms of vitamin K each day.

ALPHA-LIPOIC ACID

Alpha-lipoic acid is a very important cofactor for the production of cellular energy and helps the body to utilize glucose more efficiently. It is also a very good antioxidant and helps to rid the body of certain environmental pollutants. Most multivitamin formulas do not contain alpha-lipoic acid because it is expensive, but we recommend that you try to find one that does because this is an important nutrient. The recommended daily dose of alpha-lipoic acid in a multivitamin and mineral supplement is 20 to 50 milligrams.

CHOLINE

Choline is essential for the production of acetylcholine, an important brain neurotransmitter, and is required for the proper metabolism of fat. It is also a substance classified as a methyl donor, which makes it important in numerous metabolic processes, including detoxification; is a main component of cell membranes; and is needed for the export of fat from the liver. Your multivitamin and mineral supplement should provide a daily dose of 50 to 250 milligrams of choline.

INOSITOL

Inositol is an important component of cell membranes, promotes the export of fat from the liver, and is required for the proper function of the brain neurotransmitters acetylcholine and serotonin. Inositol is used in therapeutic dosages to treat liver disorders, depression, panic attacks, and diabetes. The recommend daily dose is 100 to 500 milligrams.

TABLE 7.1

Nutrient Dosages to Look for in a Multivitamin and Mineral Supplement

NUTRIENT	DAILY DOSAGE
Vitamins	
Vitamin A	1,000–5,000 international units (IU)
Carotenoids Beta-carotene Mixed carotenoids	 1,000–10,000 international units (IU) 1,000–10,000 international units (IU)
B vitamins Vitamin B_1 (thiamin) Vitamin B_2 (riboflavin) Vitamin B_3 (niacin) Pantothenic acid (vitamin B_5) Vitamin B_6 (pyridoxine) Vitamin B_{12} (cyanocobalamin) Biotin Folic acid (folate)	 50–100 milligrams (mg) 10–50 milligrams (mg) 25–100 milligrams (mg) 50–100 milligrams (mg) 50–100 milligrams (mg) 100–500 micrograms (mcg) 100–500 micrograms (mcg) 400–800 micrograms (mcg)
Vitamin C	500–1,000 milligrams (mg)
Bioflavonoids	100–250 milligrams (mg)

NUTRIENT	DAILY DOSAGE
Vitamin D	200–400 international units (IU)
Vitamin E	100–400 international units (IU)
Vitamin K	50–100 micrograms (mcg)
Alpha-lipoic acid	20–50 milligrams (mg)
Choline	50–250 milligrams (mg)
Inositol	100–500 milligrams (mg)
Rutin	20–100 milligrams (mg)
Minerals	
Boron	1–5 milligrams (mg)
Calcium	400–800 milligrams (mg)
Chromium	100–200 micrograms (mcg)
Iodine	150–600 micrograms (mcg)
Iron	10–15 milligrams (mg)
Magnesium	350–500 milligrams (mg)
Manganese	2–5 milligrams (mg)
Molybdenum	200–500 micrograms (mcg)
Potassium	25–100 milligrams (mg)
Selenium	30–200 micrograms (mcg)
Zinc	10–30 milligrams (mg)

BORON

Boron is necessary for the building of healthy bone. Because of rampant mineral depletion in the soil used to grow food, the boron present in plant foods may not be adequate. Your multivitamin and mineral supplement should provide 1 to 5 milligrams of boron daily.

CALCIUM

Your body contains more calcium than any other mineral. Most of that calcium—95 to 99 percent—makes up the solid portion of bone. (Bone is not completely solid; its interior is made up of soft marrow, which makes immune cells, red blood cells, and bone-building cells.) One to 5 percent of your body's calcium participates in the reactions that cause muscle cells to contract and release, in the proper function of the nervous system, and in the clotting of blood.

A nursing mother produces, on average, a liter and a half (a little more than one and one-half quarts) of milk per day when her child is breastfeeding exclusively. That much breastmilk contains fifty grams (one and three-quarters ounces) of fat; 100 grams (three and one-half ounces) of lactose, or milk sugar, which is a form of carbohydrate; and 2,000 to 3,000 milligrams of calcium. Some women worry that breastfeeding will compromise their calcium levels enough to increase their risk of developing osteoporosis. It is true that your bones give up some of their calcium stores to supply your baby with adequate calcium, no matter how much supplemental calcium you take. This appears to be a part of nature's plan that cannot be altered by even the most scientific approach to supplementation. The good news is that once you have finished nursing, your bones are built right back up. Most research on the subject indicates that your bones come back even stronger than before you breastfed! By breastfeeding, you may actually be strengthening your bones over the long term.

We do advise all women to get 400 to 1,200 milligrams of supplemental calcium each day. Calcium deficiency during pregnancy can compromise the development of baby's teeth. While breastfeeding will not cause osteoporosis, a lifetime of the standard American diet and little weight-bearing exercise (which strengthens bones as well as muscle) sets a lot of women on the path toward brittle bones long before pregnancy. A diet high in soft drinks, fat, or animal protein can cause calcium loss. Some research shows that simple sugar and the artificial sweetener aspartame increase the loss of calcium in the urine.

Many women ask whether they can use antacid tablets to supplement their calcium intake. Antacids are ineffective sources of calcium because the stomach has to be acidic for good calcium absorption, and antacids cause the stomach to become alkaline. Because they cause the stomach to become alkaline, they inhibit calcium absorption.

With calcium levels, we look for a range of 9.7 to 10.1 on the chem panel (see page 72). If a woman has been taking adequate amounts of calcium and still falls below that range, taking a hydrochloric acid (HCl) supplement may help the body assimilate the calcium. The best way to measure calcium levels is with a red blood cell (RBC) mineral test.

When choosing supplements containing calcium, it is important to pay attention to the form of calcium a product contains. We recommend a supplement that provides easy-to-absorb forms of calcium such as calcium citrate, calcium lactate, and calcium malate. *Avoid* calcium carbonate, which is the least expensive and least absorbable form of calcium. It is derived from stones and shells and it has to be ionized, or electrically charged, for absorption in the body. For that to happen, there must be plenty of HCl in the stomach, and many people do not make it in adequate amounts. (More about HCl later in this chapter.) Many calcium supplements contain calcium citrate, which is generally manufactured by putting eggshells in a vat of lemon juice. The juice pulls the calcium out of the shell and chelates (KEE-laytes), or binds, it with the citrate from the lemon. This is a form of calcium that your body can easily assimilate. Some companies make a powdered, effervescent form of calcium citrate that is very readily assimilated.

A mixed chelate including calcium citrate, calcium gluconate, calcium lactate, or calcium malate is a good choice. High doses of calcium lactate (100 milligrams per hour) are often helpful for the relief of menstrual cramps.

CHROMIUM

Chromium works closely with insulin to help blood sugar get into cells. Without chromium, insulin cannot function. Your daily multivitamin and mineral supplement should provide 100 to 200 micrograms of chromium daily. In cases of insulin resistance or other blood-sugar-regulating disorders, higher doses can often be used successfully.

IODINE

The thyroid glands add iodine to the amino acid tyrosine in order to make thyroid hormones. The recommended daily intake of iodine is 150 to 600 micrograms. If you regularly eat cold-water (marine) fish, eat seaweed, or use iodized salt, it is not necessary to have iodine included in your multivitamin and mineral supplement. An overdose of iodine can suppress the thyroid gland.

IRON

Iron is essential to form hemoglobin, the protein in red blood cells that carries oxygen throughout the body. It is also essential for the production of several brain neurotransmitters, muscle tissue, and cellular energy, and for DNA synthesis. The recommended daily intake is 10 to 15 milligrams. If present in too high a concentration, iron can become pro-oxidative and cause inflammation and free-radical production, so you should not take more than that amount unless your health-care professional is monitoring your iron levels by means of blood testing.

MAGNESIUM

Although its importance is not as widely acknowledged as that of calcium, magnesium plays a role in at least 300 different reactions at the cellular level. It works along with calcium and phosphorus to maintain bone health, as well as the health of the heart and blood vessels. Muscular relaxation, cellular energy production, fat- and protein-building, and the removal of wastes from the body all depend upon adequate magnesium levels. The enzyme delta-6-desaturase does not work to transform fats into "good" prostaglandins (see page 56) without magnesium.

During pregnancy, the likelihood of magnesium deficiency increases. An intravenous infusion of magnesium is the most effective treatment for preeclampsia and eclampsia, complications of pregnancy that can cause maternal or fetal death. Supplemental magnesium has proved useful in the treatment of many conditions, including asthma, depression, diabetes, fatigue, fibromyalgia, heart disease, high blood pressure, hypoglycemia, irregular heartbeat, menstrual cramps, migraine, and premenstrual syndrome (PMS). Research has shown that magnesium supplements improve the ability of insulin to move glucose into cells. Restless leg syndrome, a condition characterized by uncomfortable sensations in the extremities, usually at night, or muscle cramps during pregnancy can be soothed away with a supplement containing calcium and magnesium in a 1-to-1 ratio (for example, 400 milligrams of calcium with 400 milligrams of magnesium). Magnesium supplementation may also help you sleep—take it in the evening if you have trouble winding down enough to get a good night's rest—and it helps relieve constipation.

Given that magnesium is required for more than 300 metabolic pathways, anyone with a chem screen result of anything less than 2.0 mg/dL should take magnesium supplements. It is a safe bet that you need some magnesium whether or not your levels have been tested since 75 to 95 percent of people who are tested are shown to be magnesium deficient.

As with calcium, the form of magnesium you take is important. We recommend taking 350 to 500 milligrams of magnesium citrate, magnesium glycinate, or magnesium aspartate daily. The advantage of the glycinate form of magnesium is that it also helps the phase II liver detoxification pathway called amino acid conjugation. The advantage of the citrate form is that it helps the citric acid cycle produce cellular energy. There is some debate as to whether calcium and magnesium should be taken together. Intracellular testing of these two minerals shows that they both do get absorbed into the cells when ingested together. Many foods contain both of these minerals.

MANGANESE

Manganese is required for many of the body's enzyme systems, including energy metabolism, blood sugar control, and thyroid function. It is also is necessary in the production of antioxidants such as the enzyme superoxide dismutase (SOD). You should take 2 to 5 milligrams of manganese daily.

MOLYBDENUM

Molybdenum is necessary for several enzymes required in sulfur metabolism (toxic sulfite detoxification; see Chapter 3), alcohol detoxification, and uric acid formation. Your multivitamin and mineral supplement should provide 200 to 500 micrograms of molybdenum.

POTASSIUM

Potassium, like sodium and chloride, is an electrolyte that helps to conduct cellular electrical energy. It is needed for fluid balance and distribution, heart function, kidney and adrenal function, proper muscle contraction and nerve conduction, energy production, and the maintenance of a normal acid/alkaline balance. Potassium is often needed to balance out the excessive amounts of sodium we get from the salt added to most prepared foods. There is plenty of potassium in fresh fruits and vegetables. Unfortunately, few people eat enough of these potassium-rich foods. A daily dose of 25 to 100 milligrams is recommended.

SELENIUM

Selenium works along with vitamin E to produce an important antioxidant enzyme called *glutathione peroxidase*. Glutathione peroxidase protects the liver against the free radicals produced during detoxification, as well as providing protection against free-radical damage throughout your body. Selenium also supports immune function and the metabolism of some of the essential amino acids. It helps protect the body against toxic heavy metals (such as lead). Some research indicates that selenium and vitamin E supplementation during pregnancy can protect against cere-bral palsy.

We recommend taking 30 to 200 micrograms of selenium daily. This is especially important if you have been prescribed the synthetic thyroid hormone levothyroxine (also sold under the brand names Levoxyl and Synthroid). Levothyroxine is a pharmaceutical form of thyroxine (T_4). The body requires selenium to convert T_4 to the more active form of thyroid hormone, triidothronine (T_3).

ZINC

Like magnesium, zinc plays a part in many enzyme reactions throughout the body. It participates in hormone function—specifically, the activity of thymic hormones (which boost immunity), insulin, and growth hormones. Wound healing, bone-building, immune function, digestive function, and the functioning of the sebaceous (oil-producing) glands in the skin all require zinc. If you catch colds or flu easily, or have psoriasis or acne, or if wounds on your body take a long time to heal, higher doses of zinc can be helpful. The recommended daily dose is 10 to 30 milligrams. Do not take higher doses except under the supervision of a health-care professional, as too much zinc can disrupt the proper copper/zinc balance.

If you can find a good multivitamin and mineral supplement that has all the nutrients in the approximate dosages we have just recommended, you will be providing your body with most of the key nutrients it needs to optimally function on a daily basis.

Coenzyme Q_{10} Supplements

Coenzyme Q_{10} is important for cellular energy production and helps to keep the heart strong. It has also been shown to be effective in treating most forms of gum disease. This nutrient is not easily absorbed in powdered form, so it is rarely included in multivitamin and mineral supplements.

However, if you are suffering from fatigue or postpartum depression, a coenzyme Q_{10} supplement can often be very helpful for restoring energy. The usual therapeutic dose is between 30 and 100 milligrams a day. Use an oil-based supplement for better absorption.

Omega-3 Fatty Acid Supplements

The task of building a baby's body requires a large amount of essential fatty acids (EFAs). Nature ensures that the baby gets enough for normal development, even if that means depleting the mother's stores. When we see women with dry, itchy, flaky, cracked skin, the first thing we do is check her blood EFA levels, and nine times out of ten, it turns out that she is low in one or more of them. Memory problems and postpartum depression can be other good clues that EFA levels are low.

If you do not already eat cold-water (marine) fish two to three times a week, doing so will move the balance of fats in your body in the right direction. But you should not eat more fish if you already are meeting this recommendation. Due to pervasive environmental pollution, the bodies of fish have become contaminated with pollutants such as mercury and organochlorines such as polychlorinated biphenyls (PCBs), and when we eat those fish, our bodies then take in those chemical pollutants. Mercury is a known neurotoxin, meaning that it harms brain and nerve cells, and organochlorines are known carcinogens. Canned tuna contains sufficient mercury to make public health officials warn against eating more than one can per week. There are higher concentrations of contaminants in American freshwater fish than in ocean fish, and predatory fish such as sharks, swordfish, and tilefish accumulate more toxins in their bodies from eating smaller fish. Sardines and anchovies, which are low on the marine food chain, accumulate fewer toxins.

To supply your body with enough omega-3 fats without exposing yourself and your baby to dangerous toxins, we recommend an EFA supplement. We believe that every mother can benefit from the right fatty acid supplementation, whether she is about to become pregnant, pregnant, nursing, or raising her children.

CHOOSING AN OMEGA-3 EFA SUPPLEMENT

It isn't easy to choose from the enormous number of EFA supplements that line store shelves. Because the supplement industry is for the most part unregulated, the quality of EFA supplements can vary greatly. The majority of omega-3 supplements are derived from one of three sources: fish oils, algae, or flaxseeds. Fish oil and flaxseed oil are available either as softgels or liquid, while algae-derived supplements are found in pill or powder form. While flaxseeds and flaxseed oil are excellent sources of the short-chain omega-3 fat alpha-linolenic acid (ALA), most people cannot adequately convert ALA to the long-chain omega-3s, docosahexaenoic acid (DHA) and eicosapentaenoic acid (EPA). We recommend that you supplement all three.

For your ALA supplement, use a tablespoon of ground fresh organic flaxseeds in a blender drink, on cereal, or in a salad each day. (Try stirring them into a bowl of oatmeal, which is a rich source of the omega-6 fat gamma-linolenic acid [GLA].) Grind them just before using them, if possible. Do not use more than one or two tablespoons of ground flaxseeds a day. Remember, with supplemental nutrients, more is *not* better—it is *balance* we are working toward.

For the other omega-3 EFAs, choose a supplement that is labeled *pharmaceutical grade purity* and is made from 1,000 milligrams (1 gram) of fish body oils that supply 150 to 300 milligrams of DHA and 180 to 300 milligrams of EPA per day. These are natural ratios in high-quality fish oil. Fish oil supplements with different ratios are highly processed and may not provide healthy oils. Stay away from fish liver oils. These are very high in vitamin A, which can build up to toxic levels in your liver. Choose a brand that certifies that mercury and other heavy metals have been removed from the product.

To figure out how much EPA and DHA are contained in each dose, divide the number of milligrams of EPA and DHA by the number of capsules per serving. For example, if your supplement contains 360 milligrams of EPA and 300 milligrams of DHA in a daily serving of three softgels, each capsule contains 120 and 100 milligrams of each, respectively. An ideal fish oil supplement would also include lemon oil and rose-

Eileen's Story

Eileen was a mother of three. All of her children had been born within a five-year span, with her third child having been born in her twenty-fifth year. Eight years later, she came to see me, complaining of dry, cracking skin that itched unbearably. "My skin used to absolutely *glow,*" she told me, "and now it's like I have dandruff all over my body, and the itching drives me nuts. I've tried a dozen different body creams and they only give me relief for a little while. It's like a drop of water in the desert." Eileen also complained that absentmindedness had set in since she had had her kids. "I thought it was sleeplessness that made me so goofy, but now even my youngest sleeps through the night, and I still feel like I can't remember half the things I have to remember day to day."

I ordered a blood fatty acid analysis for Eileen. The test results revealed that her body was very deficient in the omega-3 oils DHA and EPA, along with the omega-6 oil GLA. I advised her to supplement these fatty acids in therapeutic doses, and to add salmon and flaxseeds to her diet. Within six weeks, Eileen was happy to report that her skin problems had completely resolved and her memory had vastly improved.

—D.R.

mary oil for their antioxidant effects and flavor, some ascorbyl palmitate (another antioxidant), and at least 5 international units of vitamin E in mixed tocopherol form to prevent spoilage.

Once you have purchased an omega-3 supplement, break open a softgel or capsule and take a look at the oil inside. It should be pale yellow and clear, and it should not smell overly fishy. A bitter taste after you take the supplement indicates that the oils are rancid. Return them to the store, get your money back, and try a different kind.

CHOOSING AN OMEGA-6 EFA SUPPLEMENT

Supplementation of omega-6 oils is a controversial topic. Most people living in developed countries get far too much omega-6 in their diets. Why, then, should we use additional omega-6 fats to encourage a state of balanced health?

We certainly do not advocate adding more corn, safflower, soybean, or sunflower oil to your diet. These are sources of linoleic acid (LA). Gamma-linolenic acid (GLA) is made from LA in the body with the help of the enzyme delta-6-desaturase. GLA then becomes the compound dihomogammalinolenic acid (DHGLA), from which the important anti-inflammatory and mood-regulating prostaglandin E_1 (PGE_1) is made.

As discussed in Chapter 3, the activity of delta-6-desaturase is inhibited by trans fats from hydrogenated oils, excessive alcohol consumption, high stress, and excessive consumption of saturated fats and refined carbohydrates. Besides these factors that inhibit this enzyme, delta-6-desaturase requires adequate levels of vitamins B_3, B_6, and C, and the minerals magnesium and zinc, in order to function. Many people are deficient in these cofactors. As a result, the transformation of LA to GLA does not happen efficiently, so, ultimately, PGE_1 is not produced adequately. GLA itself is found in very few food sources, so taking supplemental GLA gives the body an additional source of this raw material from which to make PGE_1. We recommend using GLA omega-6 supplements from black currant seed or borage oils. Evening primrose oil is a popular omega-6 supplement, but it contains mostly LA and a very small amount of GLA when compared with black currant seed or borage oil.

Also discussed in Chapter 3 was the fact that DHGLA can be transformed either into "good" prostaglandins or into another fat, arachidonic acid (AA). If DHGLA goes into the AA pathway, only the "bad" prostaglandin E_2 (PGE_2) and compounds known as leukotrienes will be the end result. The activity of an enzyme called delta-5-desaturase determines which direction the DHGLA will take. Insulin increases delta-5-desaturase activity, channeling more DHGLA into the production of the undesirable AA and less into the beneficial PGE_1. This helps to explain why high blood insulin levels wreak such havoc in the body. If insulin resistance (see page 103) and high insulin levels develop, delta-5-desaturase works overtime and very little PGE_1 is formed. Individuals with insulin resistance or diabetes can benefit greatly from GLA supplementation. To decrease delta-5-desaturase activity, your body needs adequate omega-3 oils, as well as vitamin C, zinc, and the B vitamin niacin.

If you suffer from inflammation, skin rashes, or muscle cramping, a 100-milligram daily dose of GLA may help.

Blood-Sugar Control: Chromium and Vanadium Supplements

Your body uses the mineral chromium, along with niacin and the amino acids glycine, glutamic acid, and cysteine, to build a compound known as glucose tolerance factor (GTF). The action of insulin is strongly enhanced by GTF. Studies have linked high blood-sugar and insulin levels with chromium deficiency, and chromium supplementation has been shown to help people with diabetes maintain healthy blood-sugar levels. For some people, chromium supplements enhance weight loss.

Vanadium is an essential mineral that appears to mimic the action of insulin, supporting balanced blood-sugar levels. Studies show that taking supplements of this mineral improve the body's response to insulin.

If you have a tendency toward insulin resistance and blood-sugar imbalances, try taking 10 to 20 micrograms of vanadium along with 50 to 200 micrograms of chromium per day.

Protein Powders

There are many protein powders on the market. Most are made from soy or a milk derivative called whey. If whey powders are well digested and you have no allergies to these ingredients, they can be good sources of protein. There is growing evidence that soy protein is not beneficial for numerous reasons, among the most important of which are that it can add too many estrogenlike compounds to the body and that it limits mineral absorption. If you experience significant anxiety, depression, insomnia, panic attacks, or other signs of serious neurotransmitter imbalance, a customized pharmaceutical-grade amino acid powder based upon specific laboratory test results often yields the best results. (More about amino acid analysis below.)

Assessing Supplement
Needs with Lab Tests

Specific laboratory tests can be used to evaluate the body's levels of and requirements for specific nutrients. Such tests allow for targeted supplementation for people who need more of a boost than a general supplement plan can give them. It is best to find a practitioner of clinical nutrition to administer these tests, design a supplement plan based on the results, and help you to adjust to the new regimen. Let us look at some of the most useful of these tests, and what they can show.

AMINO ACID ANALYSIS

When you eat a food that contains protein, your body breaks it down into amino acids, which can then be used to make energy or to build tissues or to make body chemicals such as enzymes and neurotransmitters. Many different health problems may be caused by amino acid deficiencies, including alcoholism; anxiety; cardiovascular disease; chemical sensitivities; depression; dermatitis; eye disorders; free-radical stress; high cholesterol and triglyceride levels; high blood pressure; inflammatory illnesses such as allergies, asthma, or rheumatoid arthritis; insomnia; liver detoxification problems; panic attacks; poor immunity; poor wound healing; and seizures. In infants and children, neural tube defects and behavior problems have been linked to a lack of amino acids.

Many women who are prescribed fluoxetine (Prozac) or other selective serotonin reuptake inhibitors (SSRIs) for postpartum depression have low levels of the amino acid required for the brain to make serotonin. The body needs the amino-acid compound 5-hydroxy-tryptophan and pyridoxal5-phosphate (P5P), the active form of vitamin B_6, to build this neurotransmitter. Mild to moderate cases of depression are often dramatically helped by providing these two precursors, along with essential fatty acids. A shortage of the amino acid tyrosine, the basic building block of thyroid hormones and the adrenal catecholamines, can significantly contribute to depression, postpartum fatigue, or weight gain, because it is also the precursor for the brain neurotransmitters norepinephrine, epinephrine, and dopamine. A typical supplement regimen for replenishing serotonin and catecholamine levels is 1,000 milligrams of tyrosine three times a day, 300 milligrams of 5-HTP three times a day, and 50 to 75 milligrams of P5P daily, along with 800 micrograms of folic acid. If epinephrine (adrenaline) levels are low, 750 milligrams of the amino acid cysteine, along with 100 micrograms each of selenium and folic acid, are often needed.

Amino acid imbalances can be measured through blood or urine tests. There is even a laboratory test that can measure your amino acid levels by a simple finger prick blood test that you can do at home. (See the Resources section at the end of this book for more information.)

If most of the amino acids on an individual's amino acid profile are low, she is either not taking in adequate protein or is not digesting or absorbing the protein that she does eat. If scores on the profile are low despite adequate protein intake, we look at digestive function. Does the person make enough digestive enzymes to break proteins down into amino acids? If not, the proteins cannot be well absorbed into the body through the intestinal wall. In such cases, the simple addition of appropriate digestive enzymes often enables the body to obtain adequate amounts of amino acids from food again. In cases of severe amino acid imbalance, especially with people who are suffering from anxiety, chronic insomnia, or mood swings, a precise custom-blended amino acid formulation can be prescribed. Many compounding pharmacists can fill this type of prescription. There are laboratories that specialize in making pharmaceutical-grade amino acid powders based upon submitted lab tests. (See the Resources section at the end of this book for more information.) These customized amino acid powders work for a fairly high percentage of people and often correct imbalances in people who thought their only option was to take SSRIs. In many cases, taking extra doses of 5-HTP, tyrosine, and P5P three to four times a day can completely eliminate depression caused by serotonin and catecholamine deficiencies and imbalances.

Kathy's Story

During her first consultation, Kathy told me that she had been feeling depressed and anxious since her son's birth ten years earlier. Her husband had divorced her, having grown tired of her melancholy moods and lack of enthusiasm for life. As a working single mother, Kathy found that it took all of her energy just to get out of bed in the morning, make breakfast for her son, take him to school, and go to work. She complained of being tired all the time but being unable to sleep.

Her previous doctor had put her on antidepressants, which she hadn't liked at all. She claimed they had given her facial tics and muscle spasms, and that they had made her feel numb and distant from others. I suspected that her stores of protein-building blocks—the amino acids—might be low. I ran a test called a blood amino acid profile and found that she was severely deficient in the amino acids glutamine, taurine, tryptophan, and tyrosine. These amino acids are needed to build brain neurotransmitters that powerfully affect mood.

I prescribed a custom-designed amino acid powder, along with tyrosine and 5-HTP, based upon the results of Kathy's test, to replenish and balance her amino acid reserves, along with a digestive enzyme supplement to help her digest the protein she was eating. With these amino acids and enzymes, a few other nutrients, and a few simple changes in her diet, Kathy's depression lifted within six weeks and she was soon sleeping through the night for the first time in ten years.

—D.R.

However, anyone who is deeply depressed, having thoughts of suicide, or experiencing any other serious psychological symptoms should see a qualified physician immediately.

NEUROTRANSMITTER ANALYSIS

For many people with anxiety, depression, insomnia, or obesity, it is helpful to measure the exact amounts of the neurotransmitters serotonin, norepinephrine, epinephrine, and dopamine. It is often useful to measure levels of other neurotransmitters, such as GABA and dopamine, as well. These neurotransmitters can be measured either by blood tests to assess the levels of the neurotransmitters themselves or through less expensive urine tests. This is the *minimum* testing that should be done and interpreted by a doctor experienced in correlating test results with symptoms. We do not consider it sound medical practice to prescribe SSRI drugs without doing neurotransmitter testing. This information allows a qualified health-care practitioner to precisely prescribe the amounts of precursor amino acids, vitamins, and minerals a patient needs to help balance neurotransmitter levels.

MINERAL LEVEL TESTING

The clinical significance of the levels of minerals in the blood, urine, and hair has been studied for more than three decades. Minerals are important cofactors for most of the enzyme reactions in the body that govern cellular processes. For example, magnesium and zinc are necessary for literally hundreds of metabolic pathways in the body to run smoothly. Deficiencies of any of the other important minerals the body needs can trigger multiple disease processes.

The measurement of toxic heavy metals such as aluminum, antimony, arsenic, cadmium, lead, mercury, nickel, and uranium is also useful. These heavy metals occur naturally, but since the advent of industrialization, they have been dumped in large amounts into the environment as wastes. Heavy metals stress the detoxification organs and act as catalysts that speed up the production of free radicals. Many disease processes have been linked to an excess of heavy metals. For example, high body mercury concentrations are known to be a causative factor in damage to the heart, kidneys, liver, and nervous system.

Mineral analysis can be performed on blood, hair, or urine samples. Each of these tissue samples has advantages and disadvantages. Blood samples give information about what minerals the body has absorbed in the past few hours or days. We can test red blood cell mineral levels or mineral levels in the bloodstream outside of red blood cells. These levels can be quite different. Knowing what minerals are actually getting inside the cells is important for assessing many health conditions, and so the erythrocyte (red blood cell) level test is preferable if you can get it. A regular blood chemistry will test serum levels—the amount of minerals found in the watery part of the blood. A sample blood mineral test result appears on page 279.

Urine mineral analysis reveals which minerals the body is getting rid of, providing useful information about recent exposure to toxic metals. If a person is carrying a high toxic mineral load, a qualified physician can perform a procedure called *chelation,* in which a compound that draws out heavy metals is injected into the bloodstream and binds chemically to those heavy metals. Once it has done so, the metals can be flushed away in the urine. A sample of a urine mineral analysis can be found on page 280.

We do not advise undergoing chelation treatments while you are pregnant or nursing. However, if tests show you have high levels of toxic metals in your body, chelation is a good idea once you have stopped nursing, as long as you are under the care of a qualified physician.

Hair analysis is useful for identifying long-term exposures to toxic metals and for the evaluation of long-standing mineral imbalances. In the past, many hair mineral analysis tests had problems with accuracy. The accuracy of the tests has now been greatly improved by many labs. The hair sample used must be free of chemicals from shampoos, conditioners, sprays, and dyes, which can change the results. The best bet for a clean test is to use pubic hair. A sample of a hair mineral analysis appears on page 281.

ANTIOXIDANT AND LIPID PEROXIDE TESTING

In the process of producing the energy that powers your cells and fights infection, your body makes waste products called free radicals, which cause oxidation in the body—a process similar to the rusting of metal. If the free radicals are not disposed of effectively, or if their levels become too high, they can damage the body. Antioxidants, substances that neutralize free radicals, are both made within the cells and supplied through the foods we eat. Because stressful modern lifestyles, poor diet, depleted foods, and environmental toxins all conspire to increase free radicals and, therefore, the need for antioxidants, both antioxidant-rich foods and antioxidant supplements are usually necessary to meet this need.

If a person is antioxidant deficient, excess free radicals break down the fats that make up cell membranes, leading to the formation of compounds known as *lipid peroxides*. One test that can be used to assess an individual's degree of free radical stress measures levels of these lipid peroxides. Levels of antioxidant nutrients, such as vitamins A, C, and E and beta-carotene, can also be measured. If necessary, we can measure levels of the minerals copper, iron, manganese, selenium, and zinc, all of which participate in antioxidant reactions within the cells. Measurement of the activity of antioxidant enzymes—the antioxidant substances made by our cells—gives yet more information about free-radical stress and a person's need for antioxidants.

ORGANIC ACID TESTING

The category of compounds called organic acids provides functional markers for the metabolic effects of vitamin deficiencies, toxic exposure, neurotransmitter activity, energy production, carbohydrate metabolism, fatty acid metabolism, B-complex vitamin markers, detoxification indicators, and intestinal bacterial overgrowth. This urine test can provide a wealth of information to assist a doctor in prescribing the precise nutrients an individual needs to improve her health. A sample organic acid test result can be seen on page 282.

Making Nutrient Supplementation a Part of Your Life

The supplements recommended in this chapter will provide you with an excellent basic nutrient support system. In the chapters to come, you will find out more about supplements that help to strengthen the immune system and support good digestive function—supplements that you may need in the short term, but need not use once you regain a state of glowing good health.

Some people initially complain that it is too much trouble for them to take "all those pills." They may have difficulty keeping track of how many they have taken on any given day, or they do not like having to carry little vitamin bottles with them everywhere they go. The following are a couple of tips that have worked for our patients.

- *Keep your supplements in a weekly pill dispenser.* Drugstores sell medication dispensers that have separate compartments for each day of the week. Button boxes, purchased at sewing supply stores, can also be used as inexpensive nutrient organizing boxes. Simply fill the dispenser at the start of the week, and use it to help you keep track. You will need to leave your EFA supplements out of the dispenser, however, since they must be refrigerated.

- *Write up a chart of your daily supplement regimen.* Post it on your refrigerator, inside a cabinet door, or in your button box, and attach a pen or pencil to the list for easy record-keeping. Then all you need to do is place a checkmark or X in the blank each time you take the supplement. Figure 7.1 is a sample of a simple supplement chart.

Devise your own system if neither of these methods works for you. The most important thing is for you to be consistent with your supplement program, and to be attentive to how your body responds.

	MONDAY	TUESDAY	WEDNESDAY	THURSDAY	FRIDAY	SATURDAY	SUNDAY
Multivitamin and mineral	XXX	XXX	XXX	XXX	XXX	XXX	XXX
Calcium	X	X	X	X	X	X	X
Magnesium	X	X	X	X	X	X	X
PCOs	X	X	X	X	X	X	X
Omega-3s	XX	XX	XX	XX	XX	XX	XX

Figure 7.1 Sample Supplement Chart
This completed chart shows a multivitamin and mineral supplement that is taken three times a day, calcium and magnesium supplements taken once a day at bedtime, a PCO supplement taken once a day at breakfast, and an omega-3 EFA supplement taken at breakfast and dinner.

Now that we have looked at how to feed and supplement your body to keep it in optimal health, let us turn to the health of the digestive system. Without effective digestion and absorption, your body cannot reap the benefits of even the healthiest diet or best supplement program. Eating whole foods and getting plenty of nutrients will go a long way toward maintaining a healthy digestive system, but sometimes chronic problems are created by years of poor eating habits. In the next chapter, we will explain how you can heal your digestive tract.

8

Healing Your
Digestive Tract

The foods and supplements you choose are very important parts of the big picture of good postpartum nutrition. However, if you do not efficiently digest and absorb those foods and supplements, much of their benefit can be lost. Typical conventional doctors do not think in terms of digestive health when they see people with arthritis, asthma, hay fever, persistent rashes, or other chronic conditions. However, in functional nutrition, the science of digestion, absorption, and the factor we term *gut ecology* (the number and type of beneficial bacteria in the large intestines) is very important in the treatment of many chronic disorders.

Digestive tract imbalances may show up subtly in some people, but complaints such as acid reflux, bloating, constipation, diarrhea, gas, heartburn, and indigestion are among the most common gastrointestinal (GI) complaints addressed by American physicians. More than 200 pharmaceutical agents have been designed to suppress such symptoms without healing the underlying problem. Many of the drugs used for GI problems can end up causing more difficulties than they solve, because they push the body even further away from its natural balance point. Nutrition can do what drugs cannot: give the GI tract what it needs to repair itself and restore its own ideal state of balance.

In a balanced GI tract, the stomach, pancreas, liver, and small intestine are able to make all of the enzymes and acids necessary to break foods down into their most basic components—vitamins, minerals, sugars, fatty acids, amino acids, and fiber. A balanced large intestine (colon) contains healthy populations of probiotic, or "good," bacteria and a minimum of "bad" putrefactive bacteria. Probiotics actually exist throughout much of the GI tract, keeping naturally occurring putrefactive bacteria and yeasts from becoming overgrown and releasing toxins into the body.

In this chapter, we will give you a complete program for gastrointestinal support. You will discover why eliminating certain foods from your diet may cure your asthma, eczema, or hay fever. You will find out about supplements that will help you to maintain optimal intestinal health, and about natural ways to heal bloating, constipation, gas pains, and other symptoms often lumped into the category of irritable bowel syndrome (IBS). You will learn how to enhance your body's absorption of vital nutrients throughout the digestive process with supplements that are safe both for you and for your nursing baby.

Your Digestive Tract, Start to Finish

Digestion begins before the first bite of a meal touches your lips. The smell, sight, and sound of food prompts the secretion of important hormones and hormonelike chemicals that support the digestive process. If you are stressed and rushed around mealtime, if you are dealing with guilt about poor food choices or have other unresolved issues about food, or if you have certain nutritional defiencies, those hormones and chemicals may not be made in adequate amounts to fully support good digestion. Taking time out to make meals as low-stress as possible and dealing with food issues can make a big difference in your digestive health.

Let's say you sit down to a nutritious lunch—a poached salmon fillet on a bed of spring greens, brown rice, and fresh organic tomatoes sprinkled with lightly toasted pumpkinseeds and topped with an olive oil vinaigrette. This meal is a good source of carbohydrates, protein, healthy fats, vitamins, minerals, and phytonutrients. In your mouth, chewing begins to break the food down mechanically and to mix it with saliva. Saliva contains amylase, an enzyme that breaks down carbohydrates.

The first step toward good digestion is to chew your food thoroughly. Thoroughly chewed food is already partly digested by the time it reaches the stomach. If food isn't completely broken down by the time it reaches the large intestine, the bacteria that reside there do their best to finish the job—with the unfortunate side effect of gas formation. The formation of pockets of gas in the colon can cause considerable pain, cramping, bloating, flatulence, and even diarrhea. A good rule of thumb, according to nutritional researcher and author Jeffrey Bland, Ph.D., is that if you can still identify the food in your mouth by its texture (not by its taste), you need to chew it some more.

Even a mother who has always had impeccable table manners may begin to wolf down her food after her baby arrives—mainly because she knows that she may not be able to eat much before her infant demands her attention. One new mother described a good technique for having a leisurely meal with her spouse and demanding baby:

> We take turns. . . . I nurse David before we start, and then my husband holds him right there at the table while I eat, sometimes in the baby sling or the front pack, and walks him if necessary. When I'm done, I take him and sit there or walk around near the table while my husband eats. Sometimes it takes us an hour, but being able to enjoy our food without hurrying is worth it to us.

Once your meal has been chewed and swallowed, it passes through a tube called the *esophagus* and into the stomach to be broken down further. (See Figure 8.1 for basic diagram of the parts of the digestive tract.) Specialized cells in the stomach wall called *parietal cells* make hydrochloric acid (HCl), which acts on the food. Another kind of cell in the stomach, called a *chief cell,* makes a protein-digesting enzyme called *pepsin,* which requires HCl to become activated. Gastric lipase, a fat-digesting enzyme, is also produced in the stomach. These enzymes go to work further breaking down food (especially protein and fats) into more digestible components. Rhythmic contractions of the muscular stomach walls mix and

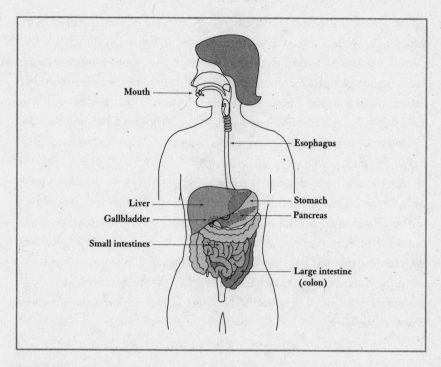

Figure 8.1 The Digestive Tract
The drawing above shows the organs and structure of the digestive tract.

mash the foods and acid to make a soupy mixture, referred to as *chyme* in medical circles.

A valve at the intersection of the stomach and small intestine is signaled to open and let the chyme through when it reaches a certain level of acidity. As chyme passes little by little into the small intestine, the pancreas secretes more digestive enzymes, including amylase (which digests starches); trypsin, chymotrypsin, elastase, and carboxypeptidase (which digest proteins); and pancreatic lipase (which digests fats). These enzymes finish the job of breaking your meal down into macronutrients—starches into carbohydrates, proteins into amino acids, and fats into fatty acids. Digestive enzymes are made from amino acids and vitamin or mineral coenzymes, including the B vitamins and the minerals iron, magnesium, manganese, selenium, and zinc. Nutrient deficiencies and chronic health conditions can both create and result from subtle enzyme deficiencies.

Bile is a fat-digesting biochemical made in the liver and stored in the gallbladder. When a meal passes into the small intestine, the gallbladder pumps bile into the mix. It works in much the same manner as soap, breaking fat globules into smaller ones that are more easily broken down further by pancreatic lipase. Bile is also important for the absorption of fat-soluble vitamins A, D, E, and K. The release of both bile and the pancreatic enzymes depends on the availability of enough hydrochloric acid in the stomach.

Once your meal has passed through the length of the small intestine, most of the nutrients have been absorbed and sent to the liver, where they are processed and sent back out into the circulation for use by cells throughout your body. What remains passes into the large intestine, or colon, which comprises the last three feet of the GI tract. There, probiotics finish breaking down any food particles that remain. Water is absorbed through the colon walls back into the body, and the remainder is expelled as a bowel movement.

Assessing the Health of the Digestive System

We can look at the function of each part of the digestive system—the stomach, the small intestine, and the large intestine (colon)—with a variety of diagnostic tests. Two of the most valuable are the comprehensive digestive stool analysis, or CDSA, and the intestinal permeability test.

With the CDSA, we can evaluate gastrointestinal symptoms such as indigestion, bloating, diarrhea, colitis, or heartburn, as well as systemic illnesses that may have gotten started in the intestine. This test gives a great deal of information about the balance of probiotic bacteria (also known as *bowel flora*) and "bad" putrefactive bacteria. It can show whether parasites have taken up residence in the colon and whether there is an overgrowth of yeasts, especially the organism *Candida albicans*. If we find parasites, there are further tests that can discern which medicines will most effectively eliminate them. The intestinal permeability test allows us to check

Janine's Story

At thirty-two years old, Janine had suffered for three years from nasal allergies, food allergies, and asthma. She would be overcome with fatigue and wheezing any time she attempted to exercise for more than ten minutes at a time, and was finding it difficult to drop the weight she'd gained with the pregnancy. Janine also had been dealing with the discomfort of chronic constipation for years.

In her initial interview, she revealed that her allergies and constipation had started after the birth of her second child. Her labor had lasted for eighteen hours and she had been exhausted for months after giving birth. "My husband wants to have another baby," she told me, "but I need to feel better before I decide to get pregnant again."

Janine's blood pressure was low, and dipped even lower when she rose from a lying-down position. The drop in blood pressure made her feel lightheaded. In a healthy person, blood pressure rises between 4 and 10 points during the transition from lying down to standing. Janine's lab tests did not show anemia or low blood volume, either of which could account for this dip in blood pressure. I then pulled out the big guns—a twenty-four hour comprehensive urine hormone test and a comprehensive digestive stool analysis with intestinal permeability to sleuth out the source of Janine's complaints.

The hormone test revealed low levels of the hormones cortisol and DHEA, both made in the adrenal glands. Janine's progesterone levels were also quite low. The stool analysis showed that her food allergies were caused by a situation known as leaky gut syndrome, in which the intestines spring tiny leaks and allow particles of foods to enter the bloodstream before they are completely broken down. Leaky gut syndrome is the initial trigger in many cases of nasal allergy, food allergies, and asthma.

I gave Janine the nutrients her adrenal glands needed to rebuild their hormone production: vitamin B_3 (niacin), pantothenic acid (also sometimes called vitamin B_5), vitamin C, evening primrose oil, zinc, and vitamin E. The making of a baby's body also requires all of these nutrients in large amounts. In addition, a mother's adrenals make huge amounts of the hormone cortisol during pregnancy and childbirth. It's no surprise, therefore, that stores of these nutrients are often depleted in women who have recently given birth. Janine also began to use small doses of natural progesterone.

To heal her leaky gut, Janine took the bioflavonoid nutrient quercetin, omega-3 oils, and the amino acid L-glutamine. She also added ground flaxseeds to her diet. Compounds in flaxseeds assist in the healing of leaky gut by providing fiber for "good" bowel bacteria to digest. Once digested, this fiber is made into the short-chain fatty acids that are the specific fuel for the cells of the large intestine. Janine's test also revealed that her body did not have enough of the good bowel flora, called bifidobacteria, that help to digest fiber, so this helpful bacteria was also supplied in supplemental form. It is very likely that the two rounds of antibiotic therapy that Janine had taken the year before had killed off this helpful form of bowel flora, which was now being replenished.

Within a week, Janine's constipation was a thing of the past, and her excess weight had already begun to fall away. Within three weeks, exercise began to feel invigorating instead of exhausting, and for the first time since the birth of her second child she could keep at it for thirty minutes straight. She no longer wheezed or felt short of breath while she exercised. Five weeks after her initial visit, her blood pressure was back to normal and she could rise from a lying-down position without becoming lightheaded.

Janine also eliminated all allergenic foods from her diet for a few weeks, eating mostly vegetables, chicken, and fish. At my suggestion, she also blended a medically based food powder into a smoothie made with juice and ground flaxseeds. She was able to add many foods back into her diet as her nasal allergies and asthma improved, but she decided to stay away from dairy, refined sugar, caffeine, and soy products—the foods that seemed to disagree with her body the most.

Within a year, Janine and her husband conceived, and the resulting baby boy was big and healthy. She was able to keep her nutrient reserves well stocked throughout the pregnancy and after the baby's birth, and mother and child are both doing well.

—D.R.

for a condition known as leaky gut syndrome. A sample CDSA test result appears on page 284.

Heartburn and Indigestion

If food stays in the stomach for too long without reaching a sufficient degree of acidity, it can be burped back up into the esophagus. The acid in the chyme then causes a burning sensation in the esophagus—commonly known as heartburn—because the esophagus is not protected by the same thick mucus lining that's found in the stomach. If you have been munching antacid tablets or taking acid-inhibitor drugs such as cimetidine (Tagamet) or ranitidine (Zantac) to control heartburn or acid reflux, you might be interested to know that the problem usually is not too much stomach acid, but too *little*. If you tend to become bloated or flatulent right after eating; have a long-lasting sense of fullness after meals; have acne, chronic yeast infections, or weak or cracked fingernails; or feel nauseated after taking supplements, you may have low stomach acid production, a condition called *hypochlorhydria*. Asthma, autoimmune diseases, chronic itching, eczema, psoriasis, and thyroid imbalances all have been associated with this problem. Hypochlorhydria can adversely affect the digestive tract in many ways. It causes the environment in the small intestines to be more alkaline, which encourages the overgrowth of "bad" bacteria there. As a result, nutrient absorption—especially of B vitamins, iron, and calcium—is decreased.

LOW STOMACH ACIDITY

If you have chronic heartburn or indigestion, you can try HCl supplements. This recommendation may seem to be the opposite of what most people are told by their physicians, so let us explain. In past decades, doctors performed tests with stomach tubes that told them if the pH (a measure of the level of acidity) in your stomach was too low or too high. Most doctors no longer obtain this essential diagnostic information because of changes in the kind of scope tube now used. Why this incredibly important diagnostic information has been left off the new generations of equipment is hard to fathom. These days, the vast majority of gastroen-terologists assume that if you have stomach symptoms like burning, that you have too much acid. They go on to prescribe powerful acid-lowering drugs without actually ascertaining whether this is the case. If these drugs are prescribed for people who don't need them, they can bring harmful effects to the whole body by interfering with the digestion of proteins and the ionization of minerals that renders them more easily absorbable. People who do not have enough HCl very often lack the amino acids needed to make adequate amounts of brain neurotransmitters and are se-riously lacking in red blood cell levels of important minerals like magne-sium. This physiologic price is far too much to pay for a lack of proper diagnosis.

If your stomach does not make enough HCl, bacteria take over the job of digestion from enzymes, causing fermentation of carbohydrates and putrefaction of proteins. Some of the byproducts of bacterial digestion are carbon dioxide gas, alcohol production, and, in the case of bacterial di-gestion of proteins, foul-smelling compounds such as indoles. If your doc-tor tells you that you need to take a powerful acid-reducing drug, please do insist on a test that does what is called a *differential diagnosis* between too much or too little stomach acid before committing yourself to such a regimen.

The lower the levels of HCl in your stomach, the thinner the protec-tive mucous lining of the stomach because it is stimulated and thickened by the presence of HCl. You can stimulate the production of this protec-tive mucous lining of the stomach by taking deglycyrrhizinated licorice (DGL) and by slowly increasing your hydrochloric acid levels as the mu-cous lining thickens. DGL is a form of licorice from which glycyrrhizinic acid, which increases blood pressure, has been removed, leaving the GI-protective ingredients behind.

You should not take HCl during an acute episode of heartburn or in-digestion, or if you have an ulcer. You should be able to get HCl (usually sold as betaine HCl) in your health food store; follow the instructions on the container. The traditional use of herbal bitters such as gentian or angostura after meals serves the same purpose, slightly enhancing the acidity of the stomach's contents and making the digestive process more thorough.

HIGH STOMACH ACIDITY

If you do have heartburn caused by excess stomach acid, you still do not need to turn to acid-blocking drugs or chewable antacids. These drugs may work well in the short-term but they can cause rebound acidity, an increase in acid levels that makes another dose of the drug necessary. They can also decrease the absorption of calcium and iron and cause constipation or diarrhea. Continually reducing the acidity of the stomach can even cause you to get more urinary tract infections, and can worsen imbalances between good and bad intestinal bacteria. Instead of using antacids, try chewing and swallowing one or two 380-milligram tablets of DGL. Sometimes, merely drinking a glass of room-temperature water is all you need to relieve acid reflux discomfort. Herbal teas such as slippery elm or meadowsweet can help, too. Or you can try drinking some fresh raw potato or cabbage juice if you have a juicer to make it with.

If you tend to have heartburn or indigestion, try a few simple lifestyle changes that are often helpful:

- Do not eat for three hours before going to bed.
- Avoid heavy, fatty, and fried foods; acidic foods like cooked tomatoes; and exceedingly spicy foods.
- Do not lie down just after eating.
- If you tend to have heartburn at night, raise the head of your bed a couple of inches with some wooden blocks under the bedframe. You won't notice the change but your stomach will.

HIATAL HERNIA

Another factor that can cause or contribute to heartburn and indigestion is a pregnancy-induced hiatal hernia. This is a condition caused by the stomach being pushed up too high within the body by the presence of the baby and not coming back down into position after delivery. If this is your problem, a qualified applied kinesiologist should be able to pull your stomach down into its proper anatomical position with a manual treatment that causes little pain and poses little difficulty. Often just one treatment is necessary to correct this condition.

DIGESTIVE ENZYME DEFICIENCY

In the days before food processing, what humans ate—especially fresh vegetables and fruits—contained enzymes that added to the effects of those made in the GI tract. Today, many of the foods we eat have been stripped or depleted of their natural enzymes by the time we consume them. Fresh papaya is a wonderful source of food-digesting enzymes, as are other raw, fresh fruits and vegetables. Be sure to eat some produce in its raw, unprocessed state to get the benefits of the enzymes it contains.

Digestive enzyme supplementation can be helpful for people with chronic digestive complaints such as gas, bloating, constipation, or diarrhea. Use a supplement that contains amylase, lactase (the enzyme that breaks down milk sugars), lipase, and protease. Some also contain enzymes that digest fiber, such as cellulase. Follow the directions on the product label. Many of the digestive-enzyme supplements that are described as plant-based products are made from *Aspergillus* mold, so if you are allergic to mold, try an animal-source enzyme product.

Leaky Gut Syndrome

The lining of a healthy small intestine, through which nutrients are absorbed into the bloodstream to circulate around the body, is selectively permeable. This means that it allows needed nutrients through but prevents potentially harmful substances from entering the bloodstream. Micronutrients—vitamins, minerals, and phytonutrients—are absorbed into the bloodstream along with macronutrients—protein, carbohydrates, and fats.

Alcohol, certain medications, intestinal parasites, and stress can erode tiny gaps into the tightly knit walls of the small intestines. Allergies to certain foods also can create leaks by irritating the intestinal walls. Whatever the initial cause, a leaky gut allows incompletely digested particles of food—and other substances not meant to be absorbed—through the intestinal walls and into the bloodstream. The immune system targets these substances as foreign invaders and mobilizes to get rid of them. As a result, the body is in a constant low-grade state of inflammation until the leaky gut problem is resolved. We have seen many patients recover from out-of-control allergies, asthma, and eczema when we showed them how to address this problem. It appears that if the immune system is constantly reacting and causing inflammation, the body's sensitivity to other allergens is greatly increased.

Leaky gut is found in people with many different disorders, including adult acne, chronic fatigue syndrome, chronic itching, eczema, psoriasis, irritable bowel syndrome (IBS) and other types of inflammatory bowel disease, autism, childhood hyperactivity, and multiple chemical sensitivity, in which exposure to common chemicals causes extreme symptoms. None of these disorders is well-understood or curable by practitioners of conventional medicine. We believe that this is because conventional medical doctors do not look at the role of digestive health or acknowledge the role of leaky gut in these conditions. Vaguer complaints of fatigue, mysterious skin rashes, poor memory, impaired thinking ability, shortness of breath, inability to tolerate exercise, and pain in the abdomen, joints, or muscles may be caused by complications of leaky gut.

Leaky gut can be diagnosed with a simple lab test called the lactulose/mannitol absorption test. Your health-care provider measures blood levels of lactulose, which is a complex sugar whose molecules are relatively large—too large, normally, to pass out of the intestines and into circulation. The higher your blood lactulose levels, the more likely it is that you have a leaky gut.

BACTERIAL IMBALANCES AND LEAKY GUT

Did you know that you harbor an entire ecosystem within your gastrointestinal tract? A whole menagerie of microorganisms resides there, and they're not just freeloaders. Some so-called friendly bacteria, or probiotics, are needed for proper digestion and absorption of the foods you eat. Other probiotics make vitamins and proteins, and still others stimulate immune function and inhibit the growth of potentially harmful microorganisms. On the other hand, bad intestinal bacteria make toxic substances that can be absorbed into the body. Some of these toxins aid in the production of carcinogens.

The balance between good and bad bacteria in your digestive tract is dictated by the quality of your diet. If you subsist on processed foods and all but avoid plant foods, bad bacteria can become overgrown in the small and large intestines. Overgrowth of these bacteria can cause leaky gut, diarrhea, constipation, chronic fatigue, muscle and joint pain, autoimmune disease, and decreased immune function. Toxins released by bad bacteria have been strongly implicated as causes of autoimmune disease. You can maintain a balance between good and bad bacteria—and heal leaky gut— by making some simple dietary changes and taking certain supplemental nutrients.

MODIFIED ELIMINATION DIET FOR FOOD ALLERGIES

The topic of food allergy is a controversial one. Most conventional doctors refuse to acknowledge that delayed hypersensitivity responses to foods— as opposed to immediate allergic reactions such as hives or wheezing— play any significant role in disease processes. In functional medicine, however, the scientific understanding of food allergy has moved the concept far beyond theory into proven fact.

A food allergy is defined, very simply, as an immune system reaction to some component of a food. This is *not* the same thing as an intolerance, such as lactose intolerance, in which the digestive enzyme needed to break down the food is not present in adequate amounts in the GI tract. We can definitively identify food allergies by means of two diagnostic tests, the

immune globulin E (IgE, an immune system protein whose release gener-
ates allergic reactions) food antibody panel radioallergosorbent test (RAST),
and the enzyme-linked immunosorbent assay (ELISA) test. These tests
can be expensive, however, and they may be hard to get if you do not have
a functional medicine physician. Even when we use lab tests to identify
food allergies, we still also prescribe an elimination diet; the test results
simply help us to target which foods should be eliminated.

The following are guidelines for a modified elimination diet for food
allergies:

- Eliminate all dairy products, including milk, cheese, and ice
  cream, from your diet. The sole exception is yogurt, which you
  may eat as long as it is unsweetened, organic, contains live bac-
  terial cultures, and you can tolerate it.
- Eliminate all soy products.
- Eliminate beef, pork, and veal, all of which can be allergenic.
  Also avoid cold cuts, hot dogs, sausages, and canned meats.
  You can continue to eat poultry, lamb, high DHA eggs, and
  cold-water fish.
- Eliminate alcohol, coffee, and other caffeine-containing drinks.
- Drink at least two quarts of filtered water each day.
- Eliminate all grains that contain gluten. This is the big one,
  and often the most difficult part of the elimination diet. Gluten
  is the protein that makes bread springy and fluffy. Carefully
  stay away from any food that contains amaranth, barley, kamut,
  oats, quinoa, rye, spelt, or wheat. Instead, eat foods containing
  arrowroot, buckwheat, tapioca, rice, or other gluten-free flours.
  Ask the clerk at your health food store if you need help finding
  acceptable foods.

So, you ask: what *can* I eat? Look again at the dietary guidelines in
Chapter 5. You should be able to stick to those guidelines while adhering
to the elimination diet.

If you can stick with this modified elimination diet for two weeks,
you may well find that many of your nagging, unexplained symptoms

clear up. The intestines heal quickly, usually within a few days to a couple of months, once irritants are removed from the diet. Some people feel so much better while on the elimination diet that they stay on it for extended periods, but for testing purposes, two to four weeks should be sufficient. Once you have been on the diet for that length of time, you can start reintroducing the foods you eliminated. Try one food at a time, so that you can easily discern your body's response to that food, and record your reactions in a notebook. For example, to test your reaction to dairy products, have a single serving of milk or cheese. To test your reaction to gluten-containing grains, eat a bowl of plain oatmeal or plain cream of wheat (without milk). To be sure you are testing only one food at a time, use the food in as pure a form as possible. For example, if you eat wheat bread, you are testing all of the ingredients in that loaf, and you won't know which ingredient caused your reaction if you have one. If you eat cream of wheat, you are consuming wheat only.

If you have any negative reaction—such as achiness, chills, diarrhea, runny nose, joint pain, gastrointestinal pains or bloating, headache, hives, rapid heartbeat, sudden drowsiness, sweating, or wheezing—to a reintroduced food, it is a good bet that you are allergic to that food and need to avoid it for a while longer. Try going two more months without that food before testing it again.

It may seem like a cruel twist of fate, but the foods you are most addicted to are the ones that are most likely to be allergenic to you. This could be due to the fact that we tend to eat the same highly refined foods day in, day out, at every meal, and our digestive systems are not designed for this. Eventually, those foods become irritants, and we need to avoid them for a while. You will most likely be able to add those foods back into your diet eventually, but not every day, and certainly not at every meal.

This may seem far too complicated a venture for a woman whose every waking moment is devoted to tending to the needs of others (otherwise known as a mother). You will undoubtedly have better success with a modified elimination diet if you undergo it with guidance from a physician who is well practiced in working with food allergies. If you want to try it on your own, and want more details, we recommend consulting

Ralph Golan's book *Optimal Wellness* (Ballantine Books, 1995). Dr. Golan is expert on the subject of elimination diets, and covers the topic extensively in his book.

There is form of allergy elimination treatment called the Nambudripad allergy elimination technique, or NAET, that is often helpful in eliminating or reducing reactions to certain foods. The treatment consists of a series of combination acupuncture and chiropractic treatments while being exposed to the offending foods. It works well for people who have sensitivities characterized by the production of immune globulin G (IgG)—delayed reaction allergies, not the immediate hive reactions caused by IgE—as long as leaky gut and low adrenal function had already been addressed and the treatment is done very carefully. Different practitioners of NAET have varied levels of skill, experience, and success, so choose one who has had success with someone you or a trusted friend knows.

SUPPLEMENTS FOR GUT HEALING

One of our favorite gut-healing nutrients is an amino acid called L-glutamine. L-glutamine makes up 60 percent of the amino acids within muscle tissue, and is the most abundant amino acid in the human body. Important for good immune function, glutamine also has an amazing protective effect on the lining of the small intestines. Studies in patients undergoing radiation and chemotherapy—medical treatments known to cause severe damage to the intestinal tract—show that those who took supplements of L-glutamine had less abdominal pain, bloating, and gas. For people with confirmed leaky gut syndrome or low levels of glutamine as shown by an amino acid test, we recommend taking 5 grams (a single teaspoon) of powdered L-glutamine daily, stirred into a small amount of water.

If you are a nursing mother, you know all about colostrum—that pale, yellowish first milk that nourished your baby during her first two or three days of life. Colostrum is full of antibodies and proteins that boost immune function and protect against the overgrowth of bad bacteria. It also contains substances called growth factors, which encourage the maturation of a baby's naturally leaky digestive tract. The leaks are in your baby's gut to allow the absorption of antibodies and other immune factors from your milk. The growth factors in the colostrum help to knit those leaks together over time.

Thanks to the miracles of modern nutritional science, you can supplement your own diet with bovine colostrum—harvested from cows and freeze-dried. Bovine colostrum is an excellent long-term tonic that can build resistance to disease, and is a useful treatment for chronic diarrhea, chronic gastrointestinal infections, Crohn's disease, irritable bowel syndrome, stomach ulcers, and ulcerative colitis. Some women report that colostrum supplementation helps to boost their milk supplies.

Buy colostrum from cows that are free of pesticides, growth hormones, or antibiotics, and use it according to the instructions on the product label. Take it on an empty stomach. There are now companies that sell colostrum that are designed to have higher levels of anitbodies for specific organisms such as candida (yeast) and an ulcer-causing bacteria called *Helicobacter pylori* (*H. pylori*). Other forms of colostrum are made with specific immune-boosting nutrients like olive leaf extract.

The bioflavonoid quercetin also is helpful for the relief of gut inflammation caused by food allergies. The recommended daily dosage is 500 to 2,500 milligrams per day, depending on the severity of the inflammation. Quercetin combined with bromelain (an enzyme that comes from pineapple), when taken before a meal, often eliminates or reduces reactions to foods by lowering the production of the allergic chemical histamine. It is often necessary also to take supplements of essential fatty acids such as alpha-linolenic acid (ALA), gamma-linolenic acid (GLA), eicosapentaenoic acid (EPA), and docosahexaenoic acid (DHA), in addition to ensuring that there is adequate dietary fiber and good bowel flora.

Constipation, Hemorrhoids, and Other Signs of Poor Colon Function

It is well known that a fiber-rich diet helps to prevent constipation. The best way to get your fiber is from vegetables. If you find yourself constipated, try eating a big bowl of steamed vegetables before you reach for a laxative or fiber supplement. Prunes and prune juice are tried-and-true remedies for constipation. If you do in fact need to use a fiber supplement, buy plain old psyllium powder from your health food store or grind up your own flaxseeds. Add 1 to 3 tablespoons to a glass of water or juice and drink it immediately. You should also exercise regularly to help keep your bowels moving, and go when you need to go—even if you have to take your baby in there with you!

Hemorrhoids are a well-known pregnancy-related problem. For some women, hemorrhoids can linger on uncomfortably even after the baby is born, particularly if constipation is a problem. If you have this problem, try this very effective herbal remedy: Add 15 drops of geranium essential oil and 5 drops of cypress essential oil to 2 tablespoons of a pure carrier oil such as almond or apricot kernel oil. Apply this remedy topically to your hemorrhoids a few times a day, and they should diminish or disappear within two days.

Probiotic supplements are often an effective remedy for chronic constipation, chronic diarrhea, and irritable bowel syndrome. Reestablishing a healthy probiotic balance can have far-reaching effects throughout your body. Look for a refrigerated probiotic that contains both *Lactobacillus acidophilus* and *Bifidobacterium bifidus,* preferably one that also contains compounds called fructooligosaccharides (FOS), which are probiotic bacteria's favorite food. Follow the instructions on the product label. Eat yogurt that contains live cultures to further supplement your body's levels of these friendly bacteria.

Butyric acid is a short-chain fatty acid that is also one of the favorite foods of the probiotic bacteria that reside in your gut. Your body can transform dietary fiber into butyric acid (also called butyrate). Freshly ground flaxseeds are our supplement of choice for increasing butyrate levels in the GI tract.

Supplementation of the omega-3 fat eicosapentaenoic acid (EPA) and the omega-6 fat gamma-linolenic acid (GLA) has been shown to help decrease intestinal inflammation in people with Crohn's disease, an inflammatory bowel condition. When you take your fatty-acid supplements, you are improving the health of your GI tract.

Yeast Overgrowth

The probiotic bacteria in the digestive tract keep the growth of the yeast *Candida albicans* and other unwelcome inhabitants in check. When probiotic populations wane, yeasts can quickly become overgrown in the intestines. Yeasts release toxins into the gastrointestinal tract, and those toxins can be absorbed into the circulation and cause vague but troublesome symptoms throughout the body. One of the waste products of yeast called acetaldehyde interferes with the citric acid cycle (see page 38), thus decreasing cellular energy production.

If you have frequent vaginal yeast infections or thrush on your nipples, or if your baby has thrush in her mouth, chances are good that you have yeast overgrowth in your gastrointestinal tract as well. Allergies, cravings for carbohydrates, fatigue, intestinal gas and bloating, and rectal itching all can be signs of yeast overgrowth, also known as *candidiasis*. You are a more likely candidate for this problem if you eat a diet high in sugar, processed flour, and alcohol, or if you have taken many courses of antibiotics, birth control pills, or oral steroids. A CDSA test or a blood antibody test can confirm if you have yeast overgrowth. Most of the time, besides craving sweets, experiencing fatigue, and the other symptoms listed here, a person with a systemic yeast infection will also have a very noticeable white coating on her tongue.

To reverse candida overgrowth, first eliminate from your diet all refined sugars, other refined carbohydrates, dairy products, and any foods that contain yeasts or molds. These include alcohol, cheese, dried fruit, melons, peanuts, soy sauce, and vinegar. Take a probiotic supplement daily. Garlic supplements also can be helpful anti-yeast therapy.

Undecylenic acid, caprylic acid, oregano oil, and an extract from the larch tree called arabinogalactans all can be helpful to kill off yeast (check for these at your local health food store or on the Internet). A course of a pharmaceutical antifungal such as fluconazole (Diflucan) may be necessary for stubborn cases of candidiasis, although you should not take this drug if you are pregnant or nursing. Work with your health-care practitioner to determine whether this is the right solution for you.

• • •

The health of the digestive tract is of vital importance for overall health. It is reflected not just in the presence (or absence) of digestive symptoms, but can have far-reaching effects throughout the body. Fortunately, most cases of poor GI tract health and function can be turned around by eating a healthy diet, eliminating potential allergens and other troublesome foods, and using appropriate supplements.

At this point, you may be thinking, "But you can't expect me to give up ice cream and bagels forever!" Well, many people do and feel great. Others can tolerate these things in moderation. You won't need to use most of the supplements and dietary restrictions described in this chapter indefinitely. It will probably take only a few months for your GI tract to heal and regain its optimal level of function. Then you should be able to treat yourself to your favorite foods a few times a month without problems—and with the benefits of better overall health and well-being.

9

Using Hormones to Regain
Balance after Pregnancy

While very high hormone levels are normal during pregnancy, women are often unprepared for the effects of this ten-month-long hormone bath. The transition from pregnancy to postpartum is the hormonal equivalent of a wild roller-coaster ride, complete with loop-the-loops and sudden, terrifying swoops from high to low. Throughout the forty or so weeks of gestation, this proverbial roller coaster steadily climbs a very large hill. The onset of labor sends you over the top and into the truly harrowing part of the ride, and things may not even out for months or years. (Many mothers insist that this part of the ride lasts until their children are well into their twenties.)

It's truly amazing to consider that the entire process of creating a new human being is orchestrated by a body system that you cannot control and cannot feel as it does its work. This system is so delicately balanced that a variation of only a few milligrams of hormone can prevent or interrupt a pregnancy or cause premature or late delivery. Miraculously, in the vast majority of instances, everything goes smoothly and a healthy baby is born.

Postpartum, a woman's hormone levels shift into a completely new realm. Ideally, they strike a new balance that is appropriate for this stage in her life, equipping her for the tasks of breastfeeding and mothering. In many women, however, hormone levels shift into an unbalanced state, leading to anxiety, depression, and other psychological and physical problems. This state of imbalance will differ from woman to woman—not only because of large differences in hormone levels, but also because each woman's body is unique in the way it responds to those hormones.

Hormones, like every other substance in the body, are made from nutrients. A diet designed to replenish nutrients and a few key vitamin supplements is the foundation for normalizing hormone function. The nutritional plan we have outlined will do a lot for a new mother's equilibrium—even if it doesn't end the roller-coaster ride, it will give her a much higher tolerance for the twists, turns, and loops—but if her hormones remain out of balance, she may need a little extra help to regain her good health.

Most physicians do not check hormone levels in a postpartum woman, and fewer still test for nutritional status. Those who do check hormone levels and find a deficiency are likely to prescribe synthetic hormones in excessively high doses, which can virtually be counted on to cause a whole new set of problems. The failure to make the distinction between natural and synthetic hormones has a lot to do with why conventional medicine so often fails in its attempts to balance women's hormones, and why women end up having antidepressants prescribed so frequently. Later in this chapter, we'll describe the hormone tests you can use to determine whether natural hormones will help you.

Using supplements of natural hormones can correct hormone imbalances that can have powerful affects on mood and health in the postpartum months, and they will not hurt the baby if used in the correct dosages. Paying attention to hormone balance has helped many of our patients.

When it comes to pregnancy, birth, and the postpartum months, there is really no such thing as "normal." No one knows exactly why or how the great dissimilarities among women's pregnancy, birth, and postpartum experiences come about, but it is clear that each woman requires individualized attention. There is no one-size-fits-all approach to managing hormone-related complaints, just as there is no "recipe" approach to providing optimal nutrition. Keep this in mind as you learn about the hormonal changes that happen during pregnancy and postpartum.

Tasha and Lesley's Story

Tasha and Lesley have been friends since their first year of college, where they both played on the tennis team. Tasha is tall, lean, and dark, of Eastern European descent, while Lesley is small, sturdy, and fair like her British parents. They live near each other in a small Colorado town, both employed as tennis pros at a large resort. Their boyfriends proposed to them the same night and they became pregnant within a month of each other.

Tasha knew she was pregnant as soon as she began to wake up every morning incredibly sick to her stomach. Lesley, on the other hand, didn't feel nauseated at all, and didn't even realize she had missed a period; she had some light spotting, a bit less than her usual periods. A couple of weeks later, she noticed that her breasts were swollen and tender. By the time she visited the doctor, an ultrasound revealed that she was almost twelve weeks pregnant.

The friends talked with or saw each other every day—some days to commiserate, others to share their excitement. Their experiences were so different that they both worried they weren't "normal." Tasha, who had suffered from asthma and allergies in childhood, began to wheeze and sneeze anew during her second trimester. At one point, she was diagnosed with borderline gestational diabetes, which was controlled with diet. Lesley felt good except for some swelling in her ankles, aches in her pelvis, and occasional heartburn. As she neared her third trimester, however, she became so exhausted that she had to cut her hours at work in half. At that same point in her own pregnancy, Tasha began to feel energetic and happy. She didn't enjoy exercising because it made her sweat far more than it ever had, but Lesley dragged her out on daily walks in hopes of rejuvenating her own tired body.

In the third trimester, both had the typical complaints of feeling too huge, of aches and pains, of trouble finding a comfortable position for sleep. Despite the encumbrance of her big belly, Tasha couldn't seem to get enough sex, and for the first time in her life she was having multiple orgasms. She had frequent, painful Braxton-Hicks contractions (the "practice" contractions experienced by some women late in pregnancy), especially after sex. Lesley, on the other hand, didn't feel at all sexual through most of her pregnancy, and she didn't notice any Braxton-Hicks contractions.

Lesley had decided early on that she wanted to birth her baby at home with a midwife, while Tasha had chosen a conventional hospital birth. Two weeks before her due date, Tasha went into intense labor and gave birth three hours later, almost having her baby in the car on the way to the hospital. Lesley's baby came two weeks after her due date, following an eighteen-hour labor that required a transfer to the hospital because of alarming changes in the baby's heart rate during transition.

Postpartum, Lesley wanted to be up and about right away, and within a week's time she was taking her baby for walks around the block. Her milk supply was slow to come in and wasn't plentiful when it did. The midwife advised her to get more rest, take herbs, and eat leafy greens, all of which helped improve the flow of her milk. Tasha had hemorrhaged and felt much weaker, and had a pretty bad case of the "baby blues." Nursing was difficult; her baby choked and cried and her milk leaked and sprayed everywhere. She had frequent headaches and asthma attacks. Lesley's libido returned within six weeks of her baby's birth, although intercourse could be painful at times because of vaginal dryness. Tasha had no desire for sex or even physical closeness with her husband.

Each of these two women had a unique experience, and you might find that both of their journeys were quite unlike your own. The distinct response of a woman's body to her own hormones explains the wide variation between the experiences of Tasha and Lesley—and every other woman who has borne a child.

Estrogen and Progesterone

Estrogen and progesterone are the two most important and plentiful hormones of pregnancy. At the beginning of a normal menstrual cycle, the ovaries produce estrogen, which stimulates the growth of the endometrium (the lining of the uterus) in preparation for a possible pregnancy. The role of progesterone, which is released during ovulation, is to "ripen" the tissue for the arrival and implantation of the fertilized egg. If no egg is fertilized, levels of both estrogen and progesterone decrease, and the endometrium is shed in a menstrual period.

Estrogen is not a single substance, but a class of related ones. Humans make three types of estrogen: estrone, estradiol, and estriol. Each has slightly different effects on the body. There are also various types of animal estrogens, phytoestrogens (plant estrogens), and synthetic estrogens (forms not found in nature) that are made by drug companies. In addition, many pollutants and toxins have estrogenic effects, and for this reason are called *xenoestrogens*.

There is only one type of natural progesterone. It is the same molecule whether it is made in the ovary of a human or a horse. Progesterone is not found anywhere in the plant kingdom, but, like estrogen, it can be synthesized in the laboratory from extracts of some types of wild yams and soybeans. There are also synthetic progesteronelike compounds, known as progestins, that are made by drug companies. The progestin molecule has been pharmaceutically altered (so it can be patented), and it is used primarily in birth control pills and hormone replacement therapy (HRT). Progestins do not have all the benefits of natural progesterone, and all progestins have side effects that progesterone itself does not have. There is a solid body of evidence that these artificial substances, especially when combined with pharmaceutical estrogens, can cause reproductive cancers, heart disease, and stroke. Further, while progesterone is the most plentiful hormone present during the last trimester of pregnancy, exposure to progestins during pregnancy can cause birth defects.

The following is a summary of the effects and roles of estrogen and progesterone during pregnancy, childbirth, and the postpartum period.

DURING PREGNANCY

When an egg is fertilized and embeds itself in the wall of the uterus, levels of the sex hormones estrogen and progesterone are as high as they go during a normal month-long menstrual cycle. At this time, estrogen has been stimulating the buildup of the uterine lining, piecing together the beginnings of the placenta, while progesterone has encouraged the further preparation of the uterus for pregnancy following the release of the egg into the fallopian tube.

From the point of conception forward, levels of both of these hormones climb continuously. Both estrogen and progesterone are formed in the ovaries for the first eleven weeks of pregnancy. After that point, they are also made by the placenta. Small amounts of estrogen and progesterone are made by the adrenal glands as well. Estrogen production increases to as much as thirty times above the highest levels in nonpregnant women. The effects of estrogen during pregnancy include the following:

- It enlarges the uterus.
- It stimulates the growth of milk glands and enlarges the breasts.
- It enlarges the genitals.
- It increases blood volume by 30 percent by causing fluid retention.

Progesterone production increases as much as tenfold in the last trimester. The effects of this hormone in pregnancy include the following:

- It stimulates the growth of the placenta.
- It stimulates growth of cells that feed the tiny embryo.
- It slightly suppresses the mother's immune system to prevent it from attacking the growing baby.
- It helps to prepare the breasts for milk production.

Without these hormonal changes, your body could not accomplish the Herculean task of making and birthing a new person. This isn't the only positive aspect of high levels of these two hormones during pregnancy. Progesterone can bring about relaxed feelings of well-being—that legendary "glow" many pregnant women enjoy. (If it weren't for those warm, relaxed feelings, how many women would go back for another round after having been pregnant once already?) Sex drive and libido may be heightened during pregnancy because of hormonal changes. A woman who has never had an orgasm may have them during pregnancy.

However, because hormones are powerful substances that have far-reaching effects throughout the body, high levels can affect physical and emotional health in unexpected ways. This is especially true of estrogen and progesterone during pregnancy. Normal elevations of estrogen and progesterone in pregnancy can cause skin problems or make a woman more susceptible to bacterial or viral illnesses. It is thought that estrogen is to blame for the vomiting and nausea that plague some women throughout their pregnancies. The fluid retention caused by estrogen can make ankles puffy and painful. High estrogen and progesterone are believed to affect gum health, increasing the risk of gingivitis (gum inflammation) and tooth decay. This is why it's so important to take especially good care of your teeth and gums during pregnancy.

SETTING LABOR IN MOTION

No one knows exactly what hormonal event triggers the onset of labor. If science did unravel the mystery of the exact hormonal changes that start a normal labor, it would be the rare woman who carried her baby past her predicted due date. Obstetricians could simply give women the right hormone concoction when it was most convenient for everyone involved. Family could schedule their arrival times for the baby's day of birth. The doctor could go on vacation between scheduled deliveries and would almost never have to respond to his or her beeper in the middle of the night. As it is, though, the wondrous system for setting labor in motion cannot be reproduced, and the length of each woman's labor cannot be predicted. Expectant parents are often surprised by an early arrival, or—as is the case with most first-time parents—are forced to wait weeks more than they thought they would have to.

The most prominent theory about the hormonal changes that lead to birth involves a change in the ratio of estrogen to progesterone. Progesterone levels rise less steeply than estrogen levels from the seventh month of pregnancy forward. While estrogen causes the uterine muscles to contract, progesterone prevents them from contracting. Higher estrogen levels eventually overpower progesterone, and labor follows soon after. But there is more to it than just estrogen and progesterone.

John R. Lee, M.D., a prominent physician, pioneer in the use of natural hormones, and the authoritative source on natural progesterone, believes that it is a steep rise in another hormone, cortisol, which brings about the maturation of the baby's lungs, that precipitates labor. The cortisol occupies progesterone receptors, reducing the ability of progesterone to exert its effects. The resulting drop in the activity of progesterone and relative excess of estrogen is part of what stimulates the onset of labor.

Another hormone, oxytocin, does the actual work of causing uterine contractions. It is secreted by a part of the brain called the *neurohypophysis,* which is the posterior (back) lobe of the pituitary gland. The secretion of oxytocin, stretching of the uterus, and the downward pressure exerted on the cervix by the baby's body are thought to interact in some way to establish the rhythm of contractions during labor.

A woman given oxytocin will go into labor, but the contractions will not open the cervix to let the baby enter the birth canal if the cervix is not effaced (spread thin and softened in preparation to open during labor). Inserting a gel containing a prostaglandin, formed from fatty acids (see page 53), into the vagina will help to efface the cervix, but this does not always get labor rolling. The hormonal signal from the baby to the mother, described above, may be the missing link here.

POSTPARTUM

A new mother's estrogen levels plummet by 90 to 95 percent and her progesterone levels fall to nearly zero within forty-eight hours of giving birth. This huge shift in hormone levels can have powerful emotional repercussions, including anxiety, depression, and moodiness. Estrogen and progesterone stay low for some time, usually until the mother begins to supplement her baby's diet with solids or formula.

These hormonal changes may cause thinning of the vaginal walls and vaginal dryness that make intercourse uncomfortable or even painful. Many women have little or no interest in sex for months following pregnancy, and low levels of estrogen and progesterone hormones are probably involved.

While estrogen production from the ovaries and adrenals is quite low in the postpartum months, these organs are not your body's only source of estrogen. This hormone is also made in body fat. (This means that heavier women are likely to have more estrogen in their bodies than thin women do.) Some legumes (beans), and certain herbs contain compounds called *phytoestrogens,* which are natural plant chemicals that behave like mild es-

Mary's Story

Mary was forty-one weeks along, huge, bloated, covered with stretch marks, and very unhappy. Her midwife assured her that the baby was fine and that she was fine, and that being a week past her due date was no big deal. The problem was that Mary's parents and siblings were due to arrive in only a few days from the other coast, and she was darned if she wasn't going to have a baby to show them when they got here.

First, she tried nipple stimulation, exercise, and sex to try to start labor—all fun, but no contractions came as a result. She inserted capsules containing evening primrose oil into her vagina, which was supposed to help efface her cervix, then visited an acupuncturist for labor induction. Nothing. From there, Mary moved to herbs—pennyroyal and blue and black cohosh. She followed the midwife's instructions to the letter but, aside from the baby's gymnastics, felt not a single pinch or twang in her distended belly.

Then it was time to pull out the big guns. A friend of hers had used castor oil as a last resort and she had heard many women swear by it. Over a period of six hours, she downed four ounces of the vile, slippery stuff, two ounces at a time, in glasses of orange juice and beet juice. It gave her terrible diarrhea, but not a single contraction. Mary and her husband visited an obstetrician to make sure that the baby was doing fine, and the ultrasound showed that she was. The doctor massaged Mary's cervix to try to open it a little, then told the expectant parents to go back home and wait.

In the end, Mary's family arrived on a Monday and she spontaneously went into labor Wednesday night. She didn't give birth until 1:30 A.M. on Friday. In the end, though, she was glad that things turned out as they did, and so was her family. They got to spend some time together before she was knocked flat by the efforts of labor and birthing, and they got to witness her amazing overnight transformation from pregnant woman to new mother. In retrospect, Mary says, she realizes her family wouldn't have seen firsthand how beautiful and right a thing home birth could be if her daughter had been born before their arrival. She is glad she didn't need a medical induction, and that she and her husband just let nature take its course. It seems, Mary says, as if modern medicine—and modern women like herself—want to feel that they are in control of such situations as birth, death, and any ill that strikes in between, but one of the most enriching aspects of her birth experience was coming to accept that she was definitely *not* in the driver's seat for this part of the ride!

trogens in the body. In addition, chemicals we encounter every day—car exhaust, cleaning solvents, fertilizers, pesticides, plastics, and many others—may contain *xenoestrogens,* which are synthetic chemicals that mimic the effects of estrogen in the body. Xenoestrogens are generally weaker than the body's own estrogens, but unlike your own estrogens, they can accumulate in the body and have potent effects. Thus, you are potentially exposed to a variety of estrogens daily. There are no sources of progesterone other than the ovaries and the adrenal glands, although there are some medicinal herbs that seem to encourage the brain to stimulate some progesterone activity.

With many of the women we treat for postpartum ailments, hormone testing shows that estrogen production is not significantly low, but progesterone is bottomed out. These two hormones are meant to strike a balance; their effects are complementary. If estrogen levels overwhelm progesterone levels, symptoms of a condition known as *estrogen dominance* can result. This imbalance, first described by Dr. John Lee, can cause a wide range of symptoms, including anxiety, depression, fatigue, foggy thinking, insomnia, irritability, and weight gain. An estrogen/progesterone imbalance can also disrupt the function of thyroid hormones and of cortisol, which is produced by the adrenal glands. A course of supplemental natural progesterone can correct this imbalance, as you will see later in this chapter.

Other Hormones

While the reproductive hormones estrogen and progesterone are the primary hormones of pregnancy, other hormones also have an important effect on the health and well-being of both mother and baby, especially postpartum. These include hormones produced by the adrenal glands, thyroid gland, pancreas, and pituitary gland. Let us look at each of these in turn.

ADRENAL HORMONES
The adrenal glands, one of which is situated atop each kidney, are made up of two different kinds of tissue, called the *adrenal cortex* and *adrenal*

medulla, respectively. These two aspects of the adrenals produce two markedly different types of hormones. The adrenal cortex makes three types of hormones:

1. The glucocorticoids cortisol and cortisone;
2. The mineralocorticoid aldosterone; and
3. The 17-ketosteroids, which include dehydroepiandrosterone (DHEA), and small amounts of the reproductive hormones.

The adrenal medulla makes the catecholamines—epinephrine, norepinephrine, and dopamine—which are neurotransmitters that have profound effects on mood, energy, and many physiological processes, such as blood pressure and how much blood the heart pumps per beat.

Cortisol

Cortisol is commonly referred to as a *stress hormone* because cortisol levels climb when energy and resources are required for quick responses to stressful situations. During times of stress, cortisol causes blood sugar and blood pressure to rise. More blood is moved through the body to supply greater amounts of cellular fuel. Cortisol encourages the storage of fat and the use of fast-burning carbohydrates for fuel. Increased energy and alertness—which can go overboard into nervousness, irritability, and anxiety in some people—are other signs that cortisol is on the upswing.

High cortisol levels serve the purpose of ensuring that the mother's body and the body of her baby get all of the resources they need up until the time of birth. It probably also helps to prepare the mother's body for the challenges of the birth process itself, and may contribute to that burst of energy that supports a woman's nest-feathering efforts in the last three months of pregnancy. And, as mentioned earlier, it is the steep rise in cortisol shortly before the onset of labor that matures the baby's lungs and probably has to do with stimulating labor.

The production of cortisol in the adrenal glands is stimulated by the release of another hormone, corticotropin-releasing hormone (CRH), from a part of the brain called the *hypothalamus.* During the third trimester, the production of CRH is taken over by the placenta. This suppresses its production in the adrenal glands. During labor and birth, cortisol production peaks. Once the third stage of labor (the birth of the placenta) is past, CRH levels plummet. It may take some time to get CRH levels back up to normal after this. Very low levels of CRH are seen in some people with clinical depression, so this could be one factor in postpartum depression or in the milder state of "baby blues." It may be that women who do not get depressed following the birth of a child recover their normal CRH levels more quickly. Also, progesterone is a precursor hormone for cortisol, so when progesterone levels drop, most of the time, so does cortisol. The single best way to bring cortisol levels back to normal is to rest and sleep—two natural remedies that are all too often out of the question for a new mother!

Cortisol acts as the body's natural anti-inflammatory, and helps prevent the kind of runaway immune system activity that causes autoimmune disease. In the postpartum months, women are much more vulnerable to autoimmune diseases, including rheumatoid arthritis and thyroiditis. Low cortisol levels may be the reason for this increased vulnerability. Cortisol deficiency may also be part of the reason why many women suffer flare-ups of allergies, asthma, and eczema postpartum, which are caused in part by excessive inflammation.

Dehydroepiandrosterone

Like cortisol, dehydroepiandrosterone, better known as DHEA, is made in the adrenal glands. It serves as the precursor—the raw material—for both estrogen and the male sex hormones androstenedione and testosterone. DHEA plays roles in immune function, adaptability to stress, heart function, libido, and mood. The adrenals of an infant do not make DHEA until after the child is born, which means that the mother's body has to supply enough for both of them throughout her pregnancy. After the birth of a first child, a new mother's DHEA levels are usually quite low. Your body cannot make adequate amounts of DHEA or other adrenal hormones without enough vitamin B_3 (niacin), vitamin B_6 (pyridoxine), vitamin C, pantothenic acid, manganese, zinc, and essential fatty acids.

There is evidence that women who have lower DHEA levels at the

Angelica's Story

The short version of her story, Angelica says, is that she was depressed for eleven years following her son's birth and was cured in three months by natural progesterone cream.

The longer version: She had been perfectly normal and happy with her life before her son was born. Soon after his birth, her family and friends could hardly recognize her. She actually felt she wanted to kill her child, her husband, and herself. After more than a decade on antidepressants, she went to a gynecologist for treatment of an ovarian cyst and ended up telling him her life story. He told her she probably had a progesterone deficiency.

She was stunned by this diagnosis. Angelica says she had told every doctor, psychiatrist, and nurse she had ever met that she had a feeling her problems were hormonal, but all of her blood tests kept coming back normal. Her new gynecologist suggested she try a saliva test and gave her some progesterone cream to try. This test showed that her progesterone levels were lower than those of the average postmenopausal woman! Within three days of starting the cream, Angelica started to feel normal again for the first time since her son's birth. The gynecologist recommended that she read Dr. John Lee's book *What Your Doctor May Not Tell You About Premenopause* (Warner Books, 1999) and follow the guidelines it contained. In three months she was off the antidepressants. The progesterone cream even caused the ovarian cyst to shrink from two centimeters across to almost nothing!

time they give birth have a more difficult labor. Some research points to the use of synthetic oxytocin (Pitocin), which is virtually a standard procedure in hospital maternity wards, as an additional drain on DHEA reserves. When a woman is given synthetic oxytocin during labor, or after birth to stimulate the release of the placenta, her DHEA levels spike, then fall to a level lower than that found after birth in mothers who progressed naturally through labor.

One of the most remarkable effects of taking supplemental DHEA for people who lack it is the boost it gives to feelings of well-being. In light of this fact, it makes sense that low DHEA might have some connection to postpartum depression. In some women it is the adrenal glands that become exhausted from the efforts of pregnancy and childbirth. (Remember that cortisol, another adrenal hormone, also falls to low levels in the postpartum months.) Postpartum ailments can stem from this adrenal exhaustion. Without adequate nutrition and rest, the adrenals have a hard time bouncing back.

The Catecholamines

The adrenal medulla is sympathetic nerve tissue that makes the neurotransmitters epinephrine (also known as adrenaline), norepinephrine (noradrenaline), and dopamine. These neurotransmitters have important effects on brain function, and so affect mood and energy levels. For optimum psychological and physical health, it is vitally important that levels of the adrenal catecholamines and serotonin, another neurotransmitter, be balanced. If the adrenal glands "burn out," which can happen if an individual is subjected to recurrent stress, they usually stop producing adequate amounts of epinephrine, which can cause a whole cascade of health problems.

THYROID HORMONES

The thyroid gland, located near the base of the front of the neck, makes hormones that raise or lower the metabolic rate—the rate at which your body makes energy from the foods you eat. There are two main types of thyroid hormone, triiodothyronine (designated T_3) and thyroxine (T_4). T_4 is the major hormone secreted by the thyroid gland. It is transported through the blood, mostly bound to thyroid-binding hormone and to the proteins prealbumin and albumin. Although it is an active hormone, its most important role is to be converted into T_3, which is much more active. Thyroid hormones regulate how much oxygen the cells receive, so they increase mental alertness and have potent effects on mood and energy levels. In pregnancy and during labor and birth, a woman's metabolic rate increases to meet the considerable energy needs of baby and mother. The excessive sweating many women experience during pregnancy is caused by high thyroid hormone activity.

For as many as 10 percent of all postpartum women, postpartum thyroid imbalances are at the root of their emotional and physical complaints. Imbalanced thyroid levels can also make other hormonal imbalances more severe. Symptoms of hyperthyroidism, or excessively high thyroid levels, can include hyperactivity, insomnia, intolerance to heat, and rapid heartbeat. Hypothyroidism, or abnormally low thyroid levels, can lead to clumsiness, depression, fatigue, hair loss, impaired concentration and memory, slow heartbeat, intolerance to cold, and weight gain. One study found that half of women with underactive thyroids have nightmares, while only 5.5 percent of women with normal thyroid activity had them. These symptoms can easily be mistaken for psychologically based anxiety or depression.

Thyroid expert Ridha Arem, M.D., in his book *The Thyroid Solution,* tells us that the thyroid gland is vulnerable to autoimmune attack in the months following pregnancy. According to Dr. Arem's research, postpartum thyroid imbalances fall into three general categories:

1. Thyroid hormone overproduction (hyperthyroidism) during the second and third postpartum months, followed by seven to eight months of low thyroid levels (hypothyroidism). In this scenario, an autoimmune attack on the thyroid gland first causes hormone levels to rise too high, resulting in symptoms such as hyperactivity, irritability, and weight loss. Then the damaged gland becomes unable to make enough hormone for a few months while it heals, and the result is aches and pains, dry skin, poor memory, and weight gain.
2. Hyperthyroidism only during the second and third months postpartum. This too may be due to an autoimmune attack.
3. Hypothyroidism only lasting two to three months, which may then go back to normal or which could require long-term treatment. This may be caused by stress and overall nutrient depletion, especially if stores of iodine and the amino acid tyrosine

are low. The adrenal catecholamines (see page 191) are tyrosine dependent. The thyroid hormones are also tyrosine dependent, so if you are deficient in tyrosine—which is very common— you may become deficient in both the adrenal catecholamines and thyroid hormones, leading to many mood- and energy-related symptoms.

Dr. Arem also emphasizes that the thyroid gland is highly responsive to stress and negative emotions. Women who are depressed and stressed out for other reasons may trigger a thyroid imbalance. If your symptoms didn't set in until one to two months after you gave birth, or if they became noticeably worse at that point, you should have your thyroid hormone levels measured.

Progesterone enhances the action of thyroid hormones. Women who are diagnosed with hypothyroidism may be able to regain their thyroid hormone balance with the use of supplemental progesterone. (More about this later in this chapter.)

INSULIN

Insulin is a vital hormone that is produced in the pancreas. During pregnancy, a woman's body naturally becomes slightly insulin resistant, meaning that the insulin is less effective at doing its job of bringing glucose (blood sugar) into the cells, especially in the cells that make up muscle and fat. More sugars therefore remain in the circulation. At the same time, the liver begins to make extra glucose from stored fuel, which also boosts blood sugar levels. Both of these changes are apparently designed to economize on the mother's needs for glucose to ensure that her baby gets enough.

In 2 to 3 percent of pregnant women, this natural state of insulin resistance develops into gestational diabetes. Blood sugars rise to unhealthy levels because insulin is either insufficient or unable to do the job of clearing glucose out of the circulation. Symptoms of excessive hunger and thirst, frequent vaginal infections, and frequent urination all can indicate gestational diabetes. If left untreated, this imbalance can lead to serious complications in pregnancy. Neurotransmitter tests done on women with insulin resistance often show high levels of norepinephrine and low levels of serotonin. Fortunately, as discussed in Chapters 5 and 7, gestational diabetes can often be treated with changes in diet and by taking a few supplements.

Other hormones that fluctuate during pregnancy are known to affect both the formation and the action of insulin. It may be that high levels of these hormones trigger diabetes in women who are already vulnerable to it. Gestational diabetes usually resolves on its own after the baby is born, but some women continue to be insulin resistant after giving birth. This is the source of some postpartum symptoms in women with gestational diabetes.

An insulin-balancing diet is a good idea for everyone. Type 2 diabetes, formerly known as adult-onset diabetes, is on the rise in Western nations, and the diet that prevents its development is the healthiest diet you can eat. Type 2 diabetes can often be fully resolved by returning to the appropriate weight for your height—often what you weighed in high school, assuming you were a relatively thin teenager. (See Chapter 5 to review ways to build your nutrient reserves and prevent diabetes and other diseases with diet.)

PROLACTIN AND OXYTOCIN

Prolactin is a hormone made in the pituitary gland in the brain that is best known for its role in stimulating the production of breast milk. Normally, the production of prolactin is kept low by a chemical called prolactin inhibitory factor (PIF). Throughout the time a mother breastfeeds, PIF is itself suppressed, allowing prolactin to be produced in abundance. The steep drop in progesterone that occurs during and after labor triggers this increase in prolactin production. As long as prolactin production is high, progesterone and estrogen production from the ovaries is suppressed. This is what is behind the old wives' tale that as long as you are breastfeeding exclusively and nursing on demand rather than on a set schedule, you will not ovulate and can go without birth control. (We don't know how many babies have been brought into the world by parents who believed this, but we have encountered enough of them to know that nursing is not a very reliable form of contraception!)

Another hormone, oxytocin, controls the milk ejection reflex. When your baby latches on to the nipple and begins to suck, a message travels from the breast to the brain that stimulates the secretion of oxytocin. The hormone is produced in the hypothalamus, another part of the brain, and zips through the bloodstream back to the breast, where it causes the muscular walls of the milk ducts to contract. This is the process known as *letdown*. In some women, letdown can be set in motion by the mere sound of a baby's cry.

Oxytocin also has effects on mood. Maternal instincts and feelings are brought out by this hormone. This is borne out by the fact that animals given oxytocin adopt maternal behaviors even if they have not had any young. If rats are injected with oxytocin every day for five days, blood pressure decreases by 10 to 20 points, cortisol levels drop (showing that they are less stressed), and stress is more easily withstood. Some researchers believe that the release of oxytocin even accounts for the positive feelings associated with pleasant social situations, meditation, and hypnosis.

Some women are sexually aroused by oxytocin. These women may become "turned on" while nursing and may even reach orgasm while breastfeeding. Most women who fall into this category feel terribly guilty about it, thinking that it must indicate some latent sexual desire for their babies. If this describes you, please don't worry. Your body is simply wired to respond this way to this particular hormone. Relax and enjoy it!

Regaining Hormone Balance

If you have indications that your hormones are out of balance postpartum, one of the best ways to find out for sure is to test your hormone levels. As mentioned earlier, most of the usual tests used in physicians' offices cannot pick up on your levels of "free," or bioavailable, hormones. The exceptions to this rule are the thyroid hormone test and the glucose tolerance test for insulin activity.

Ashley's Story

Ashley came to see me complaining of exhaustion, depression, insomnia, lightheadedness, and pounding headaches in her temples. She appeared pale and her shoulders were slumped. Her tongue was small and pale, her pulses weak and empty, and her blood pressure low, with further lowering and resultant dizziness when she stood up.

She told me that her neck and back had been sore since about two months after the birth of her daughter. A single mother focused entirely on her daughter's well-being, Ashley had been breastfeeding her daughter for two years and wanted to continue for another year.

I knew that the headaches were a sign of blood deficiency, and that her slumped shoulders indicated weakness in the spleen-related muscles. Muscle testing revealed further weaknesses in her adrenal, heart, kidney, and reproductive systems, and her overall muscle tone was poor. Ashley told me that she did not exercise and had eaten a vegetarian diet for years. She had not been using any supplements besides the least useful form of calcium, calcium carbonate.

During the appointment, Ashley became emotional and confessed to having feelings of wanting to physically hurt her child. She knew she would never act upon those feelings, but felt tremendously guilty nonetheless. I assured her that those feelings are common, and that they often reflect the depth of a mother's fear of *anything* bad happening to her child. I suspected that her adrenal glands were having trouble making adequate levels of norepinephrine and epinephrine, and that her brain was having trouble making enough serotonin. Production of these important mood-balancing neurotransmitters depends on having enough of the amino acids 5-hydroxytryptophan (5-HTP) and tyrosine, in addition to other vitamin cofactors.

I sent Ashley home with requisitions for a blood test and a urine test for neurotransmitter levels, plus a test kit to determine saliva hormone levels. I also had a hunch that her progesterone was very low. I told her that as soon as she submitted her hormone test, she should begin rubbing progesterone cream onto her skin each day, and keep this up until her next appointment.

At her second appointment, Ashley learned that her neurotransmitter test revealed she was very deficient in serotonin, norepinephrine, and epinephrine and her saliva test showed she had almost no progesterone. Levels of these neurotransmitters must be in balance with one another for optimal mental health. I prescribed a combination of dietary supplements: 5-hydroxytryptophan, L-tyrosine, pyridoxl-5-phosphate, and the homeopathic *Mucuna pruriens,* along with vitamin C, calcium, folic acid, and L-cysteine. These substances, when taken together, provide the brain with the raw materials it needs to restore serotonin and catecholamine levels. Muscle testing showed that the progesterone had turned Ashley's reproductive, kidney, adrenal, heart, and spleen muscles back on. I also gave her Siberian ginseng, which supports adrenal function and the immune system, and a Chinese blood-building formula called Women's Precious that contains astragalus, dong quai, angelica, polygonum, and other herbs. Because her neurotransmitters were so low, I also ordered an amino acid blood test and later had a compounding pharmacist make up a custom amino acid formula to supplement her low dietary protein intake, plus digestive enzymes to help her body access more of the protein from her vegetarian diet. I also prescribed omega-3 oils (EPA and DHA) and omega-6 oils (GLA), and extra magnesium, chromium, vanadium, and vitamin B_6, along with a high-quality multiple vitamin. Only three days after this second visit, Ashley was feeling much better, and I did some chiropractic adjustments and acupuncture to help ease her back pain. The combination of neurotransmitter precursors, progesterone, and the other natural products helped to clear up her depression and insomnia.

Scores of women like Ashley have come in and out of my practice over the years, and almost all have regained their health and energy with similar nutritional and hormonal adjustments.

—D.R.

In this section, we will tell you how to choose the right hormone tests, either through a functional medicine–oriented doctor or by mail order, and give you specific guidelines for supplementing with natural hormones, including estrogen, progesterone, and cortisol.

TESTING AND BALANCING ESTROGEN, PROGESTERONE, AND CORTISOL

Estrogens, progesterone, and DHEA must be measured with either the saliva hormone radioimmunoassay (RIA, which measures the levels of these hormones in saliva), or a twenty-four-hour urine hormone test, rather than the blood tests used by conventional medicine. The saliva and urine tests give a much more accurate measure of whether a deficiency of these hormones merits further nutritional support or natural hormone supplementation. This is because blood tests measure protein-bound, inactive hormone, while the saliva and urine tests measure unbound, free, active hormone.

Depending upon test results, it may be advisable to start a course of supplemental estrogen, progesterone, and/or DHEA.

Supplementing with Natural Estrogens

If your salivary hormone tests show estrogen levels significantly below normal, and you are also experiencing estrogen deficiency symptoms such as vaginal dryness and pain during intercourse, you may want to consider using an estrogen cream designed for vaginal application. While the term *estrogen* is usually used in the singular form, there are actually three different types of this hormone made by the body: estradiol, estriol, and estrone. Estradiol is the strongest of the three; estriol is the mildest and safest estrogen for supplemental use. Your doctor can give you a prescription to be filled by a compounding pharmacist that gives you 2 to 4 milligrams of estriol per dose.

Once your menstrual cycles begin again, chances are that you will no longer need the estriol cream. The fact that you are menstruating should be an indication that you have plenty of estrogen.

Progesterone enhances the action of the body's estrogens. A course of natural progesterone may be all that's needed to increase estrogen activity and relieve vaginal dryness. Try progesterone first, and after six weeks take another saliva test to see whether it's done the job.

Supplementing with Natural Progesterone

We have seen natural progesterone help scores of women with postpartum complaints. This is especially true for women who have postpartum symptoms that last for years. While many women assume that problems with hormonal imbalance primarily mean problems with estrogen, in fact they are just as likely—if not more so—to be related to a deficiency of progesterone, which is an extraordinarily versatile hormone that has effects throughout life and throughout the body. (See The Many Roles of Progesterone on page 200.)

Even once estrogen levels return to high enough levels to start the menstrual cycle up again, a woman still may not ovulate. If the body is receiving signals that there are nutritional deficiencies or stress, it will often suppress brain signals that stimulate ovulation. This may be the body's natural way of preventing pregnancy until a woman's nutrient reserves have been replenished to at least a minimum acceptable amount. A woman may begin having periods within months after giving birth, but not ovulate with each period. If ovulation does not take place, no progesterone is made.

The best way to supplement progesterone is with natural, or bio-identical, progesterone cream. Plant sources are used to make progesterone that is identical to that made in the human body. When a cream containing progesterone is smoothed onto the skin, the hormone immediately moves into the bloodstream, increases gradually for three to five hours, and then gradually drops for three to five hours. Women who use these creams twice a day tend to have steady levels of progesterone.

Some health-care professionals use progesterone lozenges or troches (forms designed to be held against the cheek), but these can cause steep, rapid rises in progesterone levels that can contribute to hormonal imbalances. Pill forms actually deliver a much less predictable dose than creams, because as much as 80 percent of the hormone is lost in the digestive system or removed by the liver. You generally need to take 100 milligrams of oral progesterone to get a 20-milligram dose into the bloodstream, although you may get much more or much less than that, depending upon how your

The Many Roles of Progesterone

Progesterone is an extremely important, and often underappreciated, hormone that plays many roles and has many known effects throughout the body. These can be divided into three basic categories: its role in reproduction, its role as a precursor of (source material for) other hormones, and its intrinsic effects (effects that are not dependent on other factors). Progesterone's roles and effects include the following:

REPRODUCTIVE ROLES

In its role as a reproductive hormone, progesterone:

- Maintains the secretory endometrium (the lining of the uterus) for nurturing a possible fertilized egg.
- Is released from one ovary and simultaneously sends a chemical message to the other ovary not to ovulate (nature's way of making twins a rare occurrence).
- Increases libido at the time of ovulation.
- Makes the cervical mucus accessible by sperm.
- Is necessary for survival of the embryo.
- Prevents immune rejection of the developing baby, which carries the "foreign" DNA of the father.
- Is necessary for full development of the fetus throughout pregnancy.
- Facilitates the use of body fat for energy during pregnancy.
- Activates osteoblasts (bone-building cells) to increase new bone formation.
- Allows the baby to develop without secondary sexual development, because it has no effect on maleness or femaleness in the way that estrogen and testosterone do.

HORMONE PRECURSOR EFFECTS

As a source material for the production of other hormones in the body, progesterone is:

- A primary precursor for cortisol, cortisone, and all other adrenal corticosteroids, as well as mineralocorticoids like aldosterone.
- A primary precursor for estrogens.

INTRINSIC EFFECTS

In other actions throughout the body, progesterone:

- Protects against breast fibrocysts.
- Protects against endometrial, breast, ovarian, and prostate cancer.
- Normalizes blood clotting (excess estrogen causes abnormal blood clotting) and protects against strokes.
- Is a natural diuretic (excess estrogen causes water retention).
- Is a natural antidepressant and helps to relieve anxiety.
- Helps to normalize blood-sugar levels.
- Restores proper cell oxygen levels (excess estrogen depletes cell oxygen levels).
- Normalizes zinc and copper levels.
- Helps thyroid hormone function (excess estrogen interferes with thyroid hormone use).
- Helps the body to use fat for energy (excess estrogen converts food energy into fat).
- Stimulates new bone formation by the osteoblasts (reverses osteoporosis).
- Maintains normal cell membrane function.
- Restores normal sensitivity of estrogen receptors (enables the body to respond to estrogen).
- Has beneficial anti-inflammatory effects.
- Reduces the likelihood of autoimmune disorders.
- Raises body temperature.
- Helps to prevent hypertension.
- Increases the production of immune globulin E (IgE), thus helping to prevent sinus, respiratory, and vaginal infections and allergic reactions.
- Restores normal sensitivity of the brain's receptors for the neurotransmitter gamma-aminobutyric acid (GABA), which enhances sleep and relaxation.

> • Is useful in supplement form for some cases of seizure disorder (epilepsy), which implies that a deficiency may contribute to the seizures, possibly by resulting in lower levels of GABA.
> • Supplemented at physiologic doses, helps to prevents candida (yeast) infections.

digestive system and liver are functioning when you take it. The 80 milligrams that is lost is excreted, but whatever goes through the liver on the way to excretion forms metabolites, or byproducts, that can have unwanted side effects such as sleepiness and digestive bloating. In addition, taking such large doses of progesterone in pill form makes the liver detoxification pathways work harder and tends to use up valuable reserves of magnesium, vitamin B_6, antioxidants, and sulfate.

Choose a progesterone cream that contains 450 to 500 milligrams of natural progesterone per ounce, or 1.6 percent by weight and 3 percent by volume. Make sure the cream you choose contains some vitamin E, as that is needed to stabilize the progesterone. If you are breastfeeding, be sure to use a cream that contains no herbs or other hormones, so that you don't unknowingly medicate your baby. (Herbs can have potent effects, and when pregnant and breastfeeding you should only use herbs that are recommended by an experienced health-care professional. The safe use of herbs while breastfeeding will be discussed in later chapters.)

To use the cream, rub a small amount—less than a quarter-teaspoon (10 to 15 milligrams)—into the skin of your neck, chest, inner arms, inner thighs, lower abdomen, or palms of your hands. These areas are rich in blood vessels that will draw the progesterone into the circulation. If your periods have resumed, use the cream for the twelve to fourteen days of the calendar month before the anticipated start of your period and stop using it a day before you expect your period. If you are not menstruating yet, you can use the cream for three out of four weeks of the month, taking a week's break to refresh your progesterone receptors.

Please don't let your doctor put you on a progestin, or synthetic progesterone. This is the form of progesterone found in birth control pills and conventional postmenopausal hormone replacement therapy. (Medroxyprogesterone [Provera] is one of the best known of these.) Progestins cause the ovaries to stop making their own progesterone, and their use leads to moodiness and irritability for many women. Research has shown that progestins do not help relieve postpartum depression, and that they often make it worse.

Similarly, hormonal contraceptives are not beneficial for women with postpartum depression (or, really, for any women). All birth control pills and injectable hormonal birth control methods such as Depo-Provera contain progestins. Many women have had oral contraceptives or Depo-Provera prescribed for menstrual irregularities, and have been given the impression that the foreign substances these products contain are somehow serving to balance their hormones. In truth, these women are being pushed further into imbalance. Birth control pills deplete the body of vitamins B_1 (thiamin), B_2 (riboflavin), and B_6 (pyridoxine), as well as folic acid and beta-carotene. According to hormonal contraception researcher Ellen Grant, M.D., the progestins in birth control pills interfere with production of the neurotransmitter serotonin, which has effects on mood, among other things. This could be the reason that they cause depression in so many women.

Supplementing with Hydrocortisone

If your health-care professional finds that your adrenal function is low, the most basic approach for restoration is getting adequate sleep, rest, and good nutrition; supplementing with a good multivitamin, vitamin-C complex, magnesium, zinc, and some pantothenic acid; and using herbs such as licorice and Siberian ginseng.

If the basic approach doesn't work, you may need a little more help in the form of hydrocortisone. When we mention the word *hydrocortisone,* many people's eyes widen with the fear of side effects. This is because back in the 1950s, when potent synthetic cortisone drugs such as prednisone became available, doctors began using them instead of the natural glucocorticoid cortisol, also known as hydrocortisone. The synthetic cortisones are just as much of a disaster for your body as the progestins are, and you should avoid them. They can quickly cause bloating, bone loss, insomnia, stomach problems, and, sometimes, mental and emotional instability.

Further, they are synthesized from yeast and often trigger yeast infections, especially in the intestinal tract and vaginal areas. Your eyes *should* widen with fear at the thought of taking them.

In contrast, low doses of natrual hydrocortisone can be of tremendous help to a woman who is exhausted and has a chronic cortisol deficiency. Hydrocortisone is bioidentical, or exactly the same molecule, as the cortisol your own adrenal glands make, so it does not have side effects when taken, as needed, in small doses that are similar to the amount your adrenal glands would make if they weren't so tired! It is better to take small doses of this hormone than to take large doses of caffeine and sugar to try to boost your energy. Caffeine and sugar overstimulate the adrenals to make more cortisol—rather like whipping a tired horse—which has the effect of causing further depletion of both the adrenals and the nutrient reserves necessary to make more hormone. The temporary use of hydrocortisone, in contrast, can support the adrenals by taking some of the stress off them while they recover. This must go hand in glove with restoring the nutrient reserves so the adrenals can bounce back and begin manufacturing cortisol and other hormones on their own.

Women with allergies, asthma, eczema, fatigue, or autoimmune diseases that worsen after a pregnancy are the most likely candidates for cortisol supplementation. You can get supplements of this hormone, by prescription, either as generic hydrocortisone USP or as brand-name products such as Cortef or Hydrocortone. Very low doses—3.5 to 5 milligrams once or twice a day—are usually all that is needed to calm inflammatory conditions and restore energy. Such low doses are generally safe for nursing mothers who have cortisol deficiencies, and they are usually needed for only a few months at most. If you or your doctor would like to learn more about hydrocortisone, we recommend reading *Safe Uses of Cortisol* by William McK. Jefferies, M.D., FACP (Charles C. Thomas, 1996).

TESTING AND BALANCING NEUROTRANSMITTERS

Many forms of disease—including depression, anxiety, obesity, and insomnia—can be caused by imbalances in levels of neurotransmitters. A new form of urine testing now allows us to test these vitally important brain chemicals. Neurotransmitters in effect control the functioning of the entire body because they carry nerve signals throughout the brain and to the rest of the body. The hypothalamus is a part of the brain that tells the pituitary gland—sometimes referred to as the "master gland"—what hormonal signals to send so that all the other endocrine glands will know how much of their hormones to make. If the neurotransmitters are depleted, these nerve signals will be too weak or confusing, and hormonal imbalance results.

The production of the major brain neurotransmitters serotonin, norepinephrine, epinephrine, and dopamine depends on the availability of certain amino acids (particularly 5-hydroxytryptophan and tyrosine) and specific vitamin and mineral precursors. Neurotransmitter tests tell a doctor which combinations of amino acids and cofactors may be deficient, allowing him or her to prescribe the supplements needed to restore balance.

TESTING AND CORRECTING THYROID FUNCTION

A simple test of thyroid function involves taking your axillary (underarm) temperature every morning over the course of a month, just upon waking but before rising. If that temperature is consistently below 97.8°F, and you have symptoms of low thyroid function, you should seek further testing and treatment.

Thyroid hormone imbalances are a very common source of postpartum health troubles, but the typical laboratory test can miss subtle thyroid problems. Most doctors check only the level of thyroid-stimulating hormone (TSH). Made in the pituitary gland, TSH stimulates the thyroid gland to produce its hormones. In many cases, if the TSH level is less than 5.1 micro-international units per milliliter (μIU/mL), the thyroid is considered normal.

A true picture of thyroid function requires the measurement of several variables, along with a good bit of medical detective work. If TSH results come back outside of optimal ranges (described below), we measure levels of T_4 and also look at levels of T_3. The most thorough thyroid test includes testing for levels of TSH, free (unbound) T_3, reverse T_3 (an inactive form of T_3), and T_4, as well as another thyroid test, T_7, which is a different type of test for T_3. Testing all of these variables is, we believe, the only way to get a complete picture of thyroid function.

If TSH levels are lower than 0.3 or higher than 5.1, this is a good indication that thyroid problems are present. Levels over 5.1 generally mean that the pituitary gland is working overtime to try to get the thyroid to create its hormones and release them into the bloodstream, and that for some reason the thyroid is unable to respond to the pituitary gland's message. Supplemental thyroid hormones are often prescribed for high TSH. Sometimes, therapeutic dosages of tyrosine and iodine will help to induce the thyroid to make its own hormones again. In other cases, restoring balances between the brain neurotransmitters serotonin, epinephrine, norepinephrine, and dopamine can regulate the function of the thyroid as well as the function of some of the other endocrine glands. Remember that the production of both thryoid hormones and the adrenal catecholamines requires good reserves of the amino acid tyrosine.

A low TSH is considered a good sign by almost all doctors, but in my experience, low TSH can be a reflection of low pituitary gland function. I frequently find that when TSH is low, other pituitary hormones—including luteinizing hormone (LH) and follicle-stimulating hormone (FSH)—are also low. Both LH and FSH stimulate the production of the sex hormones progesterone and estrogen, so reduced function of the anterior pituitary gland can affect levels of these hormones as well. In people with extremely low TSH levels, growth hormone (GH), a hormone made by the pituitary gland, is often low. The production of GH also depends on the presence of adequate amino acid reserves.

According to functional medicine guidelines, the optimal range for TSH is 1.0 to 3.5 micrograms per deciliter (µg/dL) of blood. If a patient falls outside of this range and is having symptoms of hormonal imbalance, I perform the other thyroid tests described below. If a woman is already taking thyroid hormones, her TSH may be low; this can be a normal response to the medication or may be an indication that her thyroid hormone dosage is too high and needs to be lowered. If this is the case, usually one or more of the other thyroid tests is in the higher than normal range.

The T_4 test should yield a result within the range of 4.5 to 12 mcg/dL. The optimal T_4 range is 7.0 to 9.0. Many people who have a T_4 in the 5.0

to 6.0 range—or sometimes even in the 6.0 to 6.5 range—which is considered quite normal by most doctors, are fatigued and depressed, and respond well to measures designed to boost thyroid function. Often these people have dry skin, mild to moderately high serum total cholesterol and triglycerides, a poor HDL-to-LDL ratio, and trouble regulating their blood sugar. These are all signs of hypothyroidism.

A selenium deficiency can cause symptoms of low thyroid function. The most active form of thyroid hormone is free T_3. Less than 1 percent of the total T_3 in the body is in the free form, and approximately one-third of T_4 is converted to T_3—with the aid of selenium.

Healing thyroid dysfunction may be as simple as restocking the body's stores of the mineral iodine. You can do a simple test for iodine deficiency at home: Simply rub liquid iodine (available at drugstores or through health-care providers) into an area the size of a quarter on your abdomen. If the mark stays there for more than twenty-four hours, your body is most likely not lacking in iodine. If the iodine is absorbed quickly, keep doing this every day until it takes more than twenty-four hours for the body to absorb the iodine.

If you and your doctor determine that your thyroid function is low, you may benefit from short-term thyroid hormone supplementation. It is best to use the more natural types of thyroid hormone replacement for this purpose. This could take the form of either Armour Thyroid Tablets, which contain both T_3 and T_4, or free T_3 alone, which can be made into capsules by a compounding pharmacist. If you are allergic to pork or want to avoid it, you can substitute the synthetic thyroid hormone Thyrolar, which contains both T_3 and T_4, in a ratio similar to that in Armour Thyroid Tablets. The commonly prescribed synthetic thyroid replacement hormone levothyroxine (sold under the brand name Synthroid), contains only T_4, which must be converted into T_3 with the help of the mineral selenium before having any effect. However, the erythrocyte mineral tests that we routinely use reveal that a large percentage of people tested are selenium deficient and would therefore have trouble converting T_4 into T_3. You must also have adequate levels of DHEA to convert T_4 to T_3, so the vitamin and mineral precursors for DHEA (see page 189) must be available, too. As noted earlier, however, you may be able to correct a thyroid deficiency with natural progesterone supplementation. If your hypothyroidism is not severe and your progesterone levels are in the low or low-normal range, we recommend that you try that approach first.

If your thyroid function is found to be too high, your doctor will prescribe treatment for that. Natural progesterone can be effective for downregulating the thyroid. Other forms of treatment for severe hyperthyroidism include various drugs and, in some cases, surgical removal of part of the thyroid gland.

TESTING AND BALANCING INSULIN
AND BLOOD SUGAR

The metabolic dysglycemia test, a relatively new test for insulin insensitivity, hypoglycemia, and diabetes, tests for fasting levels of insulin and glucose, and tests levels again two hours after a sugar solution is given. The test also includes levels of other compounds, including glycosylated hemoglobin, fructosamine, cortisol, insulin-like growth factor (IGF). All of these can be done through a doctor who is familiar with functional medicine.

If your glucose tolerance test or metabolic dysglycemia test results are abnormal, you can almost always rectify the situation with the diet recommended in Chapter 5 or the supplements recommended for blood glucose control in Chapter 7.

Now that you have a better understanding of which hormones can affect your health and energy levels during and after pregnancy, and how to balance them, we will move on to the important subject of breastfeeding—an important factor in your health and well-being during the postpartum period.

10

The Breastfeeding Factor

A big part of the postpartum experience for most women is that of becoming a breastfeeding mother. Breastfeeding can simultaneously be one of the most challenging and rewarding parts of being a new mother. It both affects and is affected by your quality of life postpartum, and raises entirely new issues and concerns about how you take care of yourself. In this chapter, we will examine some of these issues, and offer advice on how to deal with some of the problems that can arise.

Using Drugs While Breastfeeding

After nine or more months of carefully avoiding so much as an aspirin, you may feel relieved at having your body back to yourself. Now, you think, if I have a headache or a cold I can take something for it. But then, as you offer your breast to your baby or pump milk for him, you are reminded that in many ways, the two of you are still sharing the same body. Virtually all foods, herbs, drugs, and hormones that enter your body have the potential to enter your breast milk and affect your baby.

Much conflicting information exists about the safety of using different medications and herbs during breastfeeding. Not long ago, new mothers were told that they must wean their babies in order to treat a health condition with drugs. Some mothers never even started to breastfeed because of medications they were told they needed during pregnancy or immediately postpartum. Today, mothers are advised to switch to formula temporarily and "pump and dump" their milk during that time if they want to continue to breastfeed after using a medication, but this is often impractical and leads to engorgement and breast infections in many women who are accustomed to nursing their babies on demand. If a baby is less than six weeks old, giving her an artificial nipple can cause her to reject the breast when it's time to go back.

Today, the typical conventional health-care model advises against the use of any and all herbs and drugs during nursing, choosing a "better safe than sorry" approach. While this approach makes good sense when the health of a baby hangs in the balance, scientific research into the effects of various drugs and herbs on the composition of mother's milk and the potential for harm to the baby now allows us to make more specific recommendations. The enormous benefits of breastfeeding over formula feeding make it worth considering even if drugs or herbs are being used to support the health of the mother.

Ideally, you will remain well enough during your breastfeeding months or years to avoid having to use prescription or over-the-counter drugs. Even if you don't, take heart: There are few drugs that you absolutely cannot take while breastfeeding. Most drugs do pass into your milk and into your baby's body, but in most instances the amount of drug that actually gets to your baby is around 1 percent of what you have taken. Most experts agree that, in almost every case, having breast milk with a minuscule amount of medication in it is better for a baby than switching to formula feeding. The general cautiousness toward drugs and nursing has much to do with the litigious age we live in; physicians and drug companies don't want to be held responsible for any harm that could come to an infant due to drug exposure.

We are certainly not encouraging you to swallow a pill for every ill you experience. It is almost always better to try nutritional, herbal, and lifestyle adjustments to allow your body to heal itself before you introduce foreign chemical substances into your body and into your milk. This is especially true during the first six weeks of your baby's life, when the cells that line her intestines are loosely knit to allow large immune system factors from your milk into her bloodstream. During these early weeks, drugs that would otherwise not pass into baby's circulation can float through easily. If at all possible, avoid taking any medications until your baby has been in the world for six weeks. If you cannot do so, you may be able to work with your doctor to time your drug dosages so that your baby's exposure is minimized.

FACTORS AFFECTING DRUG SAFETY

What makes one drug safer than another for a breastfeeding pair? Several different factors come into play here. Among them are characteristics of the drug, such as the drug's half-life, its protein-binding capacity, its lipid solubility, and its oral bioavailability.

A drug's half-life is the measure of how long the drug stays in your system. Different drugs are cleared from your body at different rates. The longer a drug lingers in your circulation before being processed by your liver and completely eliminated, the greater your baby's exposure will be through your milk. A drug with a shorter half-life is better for a nursing mother than one with a longer half-life. A drug with a longer half-life will actually build up in a baby's bloodstream over time. If a drug has a short half-life, you can schedule your dosages so that levels of the drug fall significantly in your body before your baby feeds again.

Protein-binding capacity is the degree to which the active ingredient in the drug joins with proteins in the body on a molecular level. A drug with a high protein-binding capacity—one that binds well with proteins in the mother's body—is safer, because only non-protein-bound drugs can pass into milk.

Lipid solubility is just what it sounds like: the ease with which a drug is absorbed into fats in the body. A drug that is more lipid-soluble is better absorbed into fats, so more of it can pass into a mother's milk.

A drug's oral bioavailability is its potential to be absorbed through the walls of the baby's gastrointestinal tract. This also is an important factor in the safety of a medication. Drugs with low oral bioavailability cannot pass through the intestinal walls into the baby's bloodstream, and just pass right out into the baby's diaper.

Occasional use of medications, when you really need them, should not stop you from breastfeeding your baby. If you have a chronic disease, such as rheumatoid arthritis, Graves' disease (an autoimmune disease that affects the thyroid), or epilepsy, and you have no choice but to use medications every day, you will need to work closely with your physician and your baby's pediatrician, but you should still be able to breastfeed for at least a few weeks. Even a few weeks' worth of mother's milk is better than none.

DRUGS TO AVOID

There are some drugs that should never be taken by nursing mothers. For example, absolutely *avoid* radioactive compounds while breastfeeding. Radioactive compounds are used for diagnostic testing and some treatments for serious conditions, such as Graves' disease. If you are being tested for a thyroid hormone imbalance, you may be told you need to take a test that uses radioactive iodine. The radioactive iodine can accumulate in your baby's thyroid and cause permanent damage. Tell your physician that you would prefer to skip the thyroid scan. If the test must be done, it can be performed with technetium—a radioactive compound that clears from the body within thirty hours. You can formula feed and pump and dump your breast milk for that period.

If you are tempted to indulge in marijuana while you are nursing, please don't. It will decrease your production of prolactin, which will in turn diminish your milk supply and your maternal urges. Alcohol, however, is fine—in moderation. Limit your alcohol intake to a single glass of wine or beer a day. Caffeine should not hurt your baby either, in small amounts, but if it seems to make your baby jittery, you may want to avoid it while you are nursing.

All antihistamine drugs—both prescription and over-the-counter— should be avoided during pregnancy and while nursing. Most pass readily into breast milk and show up in high concentrations in the baby's bloodstream. Avoid the following allergy-type medications (the following include both generic and popular brand names):

- Astemizole (Hismanal).
- Azatadine (Optimine, Trinalin).
- Azelastine (Astelin).
- Brompheniramine (in Allerhist, Dimetane, and others).
- Cetirizine (Zyrtec).
- Chlorpheniramine (in Chlor-Trimeton and others).
- Clemastine (Tavist).
- Cyproheptdine (Periactin).
- Dexchlorpheniramine (Mylaramine, Polaramine).
- Diphenhydramine (in Allerdryl, Benadryl, Dramamine, Dytuss, and many other over-the-counter cold and allergy products).
- Fexofenadine (Allegra).
- Loratidine (Claritin).
- Methdilazine (Tacaryl).
- Phenindamine (Nolahist).
- Promethazine (Phenergan).
- Pyrilamine.
- Trimeprazine (Temaril).
- Tripelennamine (PBZ).

Be careful to read labels of any over-the-counter medicine you choose to take; there may be an antihistamine hidden away in there—even if the medication isn't labeled as an antihistamine. Fortunately, having to forgo antihistamines rarely involves anything more than some sneezy, itchy discomfort for mom, and these discomforts usually diminish or disappear with the right nutrient and diet prescription.

Other medications and types of medications that don't mix with nursing include the following:

- Amphetamines, stimulants that are prescribed to treat attention deficit hyperactivity disorder, narcolepsy, and other conditions.

- Antithyroid drugs, used to control Graves' disease (hyperthyroidism).
- Aspirin and other salicylates. These may cause Reye's syndrome, a severe illness, if an infant with any kind of viral infection is exposed to it. Ask your pharmacist if you aren't sure whether any over-the-counter or prescription drug contains salicylates.
- Atropine, which is used to dilate the pupils during eye examinations, and to treat certain eye disorders. It is also an ingredient in a medication sometimes prescribed to relieve the discomfort of urinary tract infection.
- Bromides (for example, Bromo-Seltzer).
- Cancer chemotherapy drugs.
- Cathartic drugs, which are drugs that cause diarrhea, and are sometimes used to evacuate the colon for diagnostic testing.
- Diet drugs.
- Ergot and related compounds, which can be used to treat a variety of disorders, including migraine and cluster headaches and menopausal discomforts such as hot flashes and excessive sweating.
- Iodides.
- Mercury-based drugs.
- Metronidazole (Flagyl, Metric, Protostat), an antifungal.
- Oral anticoagulants (blood-thinners).
- Tetracycline, an antibiotic also sold under the brand name Achromycin.

Most topical medications (those applied to the skin) and inhaled medications pass into the milk in even smaller quantities than oral ones do. If you have problems with allergies, asthma, or eczema—the usual reasons for long-term use of inhaled or topical medications—we hope that you will be able to stop using these drugs once you are using our postpartum program. Eliminating food allergens and improving digestive health have cleared up these problems for many of our patients. While using the medications isn't the worst thing in the world, you are better off not needing them. Consider that inhaled steroids, used for years at a time, cause bones to thin and increase the risk of developing osteoporosis later in life and also increase the risk of developing glaucoma. Quick-acting bronchodilating asthma inhalers may relieve attacks in the short term, but, according to the U.S. Centers for Disease Control and Prevention (CDC), if used too often, especially over long periods of time, can lead to worsening of the disease and even increase your risk of dying of asthma.

DRUGS THAT MAY BE UNSAFE

It is common sense to avoid taking several medications at once while you are breastfeeding. If you use more than one medication at a time and your baby develops symptoms that you think might be related to the drugs, you will not be able to tell which drug is affecting her. Once you combine more than two drugs, the side effects can be unpredictable and may include problems not noted on a patient information insert. This applies to both pharmaceuticals and herbs, which can be as potent as drugs. Take any new drug or herb alone for the first few days to be certain that it isn't causing problems. Stick to the lowest possible effective dose and avoid extra-strength or long-acting medications. If possible, take medications after nursing or before your baby's longest period of sleep, so that your body has time to process the drug before the next feeding.

We have already discussed some of the possible dangers of selective serotonin reuptake inhibitors (SSRIs) such as Paxil, Prozac, and Zoloft for nursing mothers. They may be linked to colic, and despite the fact that some are eliminated from the body more rapidly than others, they are all removed from the circulation relatively slowly. Because of the chemical composition of drugs that affect the central nervous system—including SSRIs, other antidepressants, and antianxiety drugs—they enter the milk in higher concentrations than other types of drugs. No research exists on the long-term nervous-system effects of these medications on babies exposed to them through their mothers' milk. Some medical organizations maintain that it is all right for nursing mothers to use SSRI antidepressants, and this approach is becoming an increasingly popular one for treating postpartum depression. We disagree. We feel that it is terribly premature and careless to widely prescribe these drugs at this time. However, there are exceptions. If you and your doctor perceive that you are in immediate and serious trouble and need quick short-term pharmaceutical help getting back on your feet, you don't necessarily have to stop breast-feeding. The benefits of nursing to your baby and to you probably out-weigh the risks of exposing your baby to SSRIs for a few weeks. If you must take SSRIs, carefully watch your baby for any signs of increased sleep-iness and consider stopping if your baby becomes so somnolent that you have to wake her up to nurse.

We advise against the use of low-dose minor tranquilizers, such as al-prazolam (Xanax), in most cases. Very little is known about the effects they can have on a baby's developing nervous system, and they are addic-tive. There are many safe natural alternatives to these drugs that can help you relax during the day and sleep at night. Calcium and magnesium, taken at bedtime, can help relax your body into sleep. Mild to moderate exercise, meditation, yoga, and deep breathing are just as effective as mi-nor tranquilizers. Herbs such as chamomile, passionflower, and valerian are safe natural relaxants that are safe for your baby.

Women who suffer from severe psychological disorders, such as suici-dal depression, obsessive-compulsive disorder (OCD), or bipolar mood disorder (manic depression), may experience a worsening of their symp-toms in the postpartum period. Such women may need medication. While research indicates that the drugs used for these disorders can be used dur-ing breastfeeding, there is no sure guarantee that they are *completely* safe. If you are extremely depressed, bipolar, or obsessive-compulsive, consult with your doctor and get a few other opinions before you give up on nurs-ing your child. We also recommend that you read Dr. Andrew L. Stoll's book, *The Omega-3 Connection* (Simon & Schuster, 2002). Dr. Stoll has done extensive research on the use of omega-3 fats for the relief of bipolar dis-order. Trying his plan is a no-risk, all-gain proposition that will actually benefit a breastfeeding baby.

Commonly used over-the-counter cough and cold medicines, decon-gestants, indigestion and diarrhea remedies, laxatives, and nonaspirin pain medications may not pose a significant danger to your nursing infant, but you probably don't really need to use them, either. In our culture, over-the-counter medications are considered to be utterly benign, but the truth is that every one of them has a long list of potential side effects, and they can be dangerous if several are taken in the wrong combination. Drugs are synthetic molecules not found in nature, and are usually harder on your detoxification systems than natural substances are. You should not be surprised if any of these drugs significantly diminishes your milk supply, either.

In most cases, you are better off finding a natural remedy for most of these complaints. Besides, such drugs provide only short-term treatment of symptoms. They do nothing to address the root issue. If you are generally healthy and well-nourished, you will not need any of these drugs.

If you do need over-the-counter temporary relief, stick with drugs that are used for babies as well as for adults. Check the shelf for baby versions of the drug you would like to use. Acetaminophen (in Tylenol and many other over-the-counter products) is your best bet for pain relief, although it is hard on the liver, so think twice—or even three times—before using it for yourself or your baby. Herbs and nutrients are better medicine than over-the-counter drugs for colds and most digestive complaints.

What if you are struck with an illness that requires antibiotic treatment? Monitor your baby carefully if you must use antibiotics. They may affect your baby's digestive function, causing diarrhea, constipation, or even colitis (a painful inflammation of the colon). If you or baby needs to take antibiotics, you can help to support baby's digestive health by giving him baby acidophilus powder. You can mix this into a bottle of expressed breastmilk or dab some onto your nipple before baby starts a nursing session. If you do need an antibiotic, your doctor will probably recommend an older drug, such as penicillin. Some women experience a decrease in milk supply with this medication.

Other drugs that are not completely off-limits during breastfeeding, but that require close observation of effects on baby's health, include the following:

- Barbiturates, a class of tranquilizer.
- Chlorpromazine (Thorazine), which is used to treat certain psychiatric disorders.
- Corticosteroids, such as prednisone (Deltasone), which are used for inflammatory conditions.

- Diuretics (water pills).
- Nalidixic acid (NegGram), an antibiotic sometimes used to treat urinary tract infections.
- Phenytoin (Dilantin), an antiseizure medication.
- Reserpine, which is used to lower blood pressure.

If you find yourself needing to take medication and are faced with admonitions from your doctor to wean your baby as a result, call your local La Leche League leader. This organization keeps up-to-date drug information that will help you to make the right choice for you and your baby. It is possible that you may come to the conclusion that nursing simply isn't possible for you. It's true that some women simply cannot breastfeed for valid medical reasons. It is your decision, after all, and only you can make it. You can still have a wonderful, nurturing relationship with your baby—it just may take a bit more effort on your part. Fortunately, too, formulas are getting better all the time. American formula manufacturers are beginning to put the omega-3 fat docosahexaenoic acid (DHA) into their products (years after European companies mandated its addition), and finding a formula with DHA in it is easier than it has ever been. For excellent information on bottle-feeding, we recommend the books on baby care and breastfeeding by pediatrician William Sears, M.D.

Even if you decide to bottle-feed, try to nurse your baby—or pump your milk and feed it to your infant by bottle, if you'd rather—for at least the first six weeks. This gives your baby the benefit of your immune factors, which can be indispensable in keeping him healthy during the early years of his life.

Using Supplemental Hormones While Breastfeeding

In Chapter 9, we recommended the use of natural progesterone cream for women with postpartum depression. Women with depression that has held on for years after giving birth seem to benefit most, but it is safe for

Holly's Story

Breastfeeding was difficult for the first few weeks after Holly's daughter was born, but she had been told to expect that. Savannah was a little bit premature and small, and didn't latch on too well in the beginning, but after a lot of trying, she and Holly were a happy nursing team. Holly wanted to go back to work part-time when the baby was three months old, and she figured she would be able to pump milk once during her five-hour afternoon shift at the store where she worked.

Holly found that being away from her baby was harder than she had expected, though, and she felt anxious and stressed from the time she left her daughter with her mother until she went back to get her. Sometimes Holly would sit in the store bathroom pumping away with her hand pump and weeping from missing the baby's mouth on her breast and her body resting in her arms. Then one day at work she started feeling what she figured was a plugged duct: a lump deep in her breast. It was tender, but it didn't slow her down much. Then, over the span of the night, Holly started to feel a deep, burning pain in that breast, and the nipple burned badly when Savannah latched on. When Holly got up in the morning, the breast was engorged, shiny, and red, and she felt like she had caught a bad case of the flu.

Holly called the nurse practitioner (NP) who worked with her obstetrician/gynecologist and asked what she should do. The NP told her it sounded like mastitis, and recommended that Holly go to bed; keep moist heat on it; keep nursing as often as she could, especially on that side; and take acetaminophen (Tylenol) or ibuprofen (Advil) for the pain if she needed to. Holly told the NP that she was in a lot of pain and wanted to know if she could get some antibiotics for it. The NP said that if Holly did everything she had been told to, she probably wouldn't need to take antibiotics. But, Holly says, she had never believed that drugs are always bad, and if there was a drug that could kill off whatever bug was infecting her breast, why not use it?

The NP said that Holly could keep nursing if she took penicillin, so she went in and got a prescription. By the time she got home, she felt so horrid she could barely stand up. She was glad to have the antibiotic. She took a pill and went to bed with Savannah, figuring she could go back to work the next day. Her husband helped her to keep the heating pad on her breast, with a wet cloth wrapped around it, through the night, and every time Savannah stirred Holly gave her that breast to nurse from.

The next day Holly felt a lot better. The swelling and pain were gone by half. She knew she should take the penicillin until it was all gone, so she kept taking it. That afternoon, when she went to pump at work, she found it hard to get much milk out. When she got home and went to nurse Savannah, the baby sucked and sucked and Holly couldn't really feel any letdown happening. She felt as if her breasts were empty. The baby got upset because she couldn't get milk into her tummy fast enough, and Holly's nipples got sore from being sucked so long and hard; Savannah wanted to feed every half-hour because she wasn't getting her fill. On top of that, after a couple of days Holly could feel a yeast infection coming on.

Holly called the NP and told her what was happening, and that she thought it must be from the medicine, but she couldn't stop taking it, could she? The NP told her not to tell the doctor this, but she thought it would be okay to quit the penicillin if Holly took really good care of herself and used some herbs to help her immune system. The NP said that she had read a study that said that penicillin doesn't even kill the bacteria that usually cause mastitis. For the yeast infection, she told Holly to take acidophilus capsules and eat organic plain yogurt, and to smear some yogurt on her nipples and her vaginal area a few times a day. Holly did exactly as the NP said. Within a day of stopping the penicillin, Holly's milk supply came back. The mastitis and the yeast infections have stayed away.

Immunity-stimulating herbs such as olive leaf and echinacea do not affect milk supply and are easier on your liver than antibiotic drugs—and they will not add to the already serious problem of bacterial resistance against antibiotics. (More about the use of herbs in Chapter 11.)

you to use even while nursing. In physiological doses, progesterone very rarely affects milk flow, and if it does, the flow returns to normal within a day or two of discontinuing it.

If vaginal dryness is a significant problem for you—as it is for many nursing mothers, due to the effects of the hormones that stimulate milk production—you might benefit from the use of a vaginal estriol cream. These creams are usually used by postmenopausal women, and must be prescribed by a physician and obtained from a compounding pharmacist.

The dosage recommended by natural hormone expert Dr. John Lee is 2 milligrams every two to three days. Do try a few different nonhormonal lubricants before you ask your doctor for estriol cream.

While you are nursing, you should stay away from other supplemental hormones, including dehydroepiandrosterone (DHEA) and melatonin. Herbal remedies can help you sleep as well as melatonin can, and if progesterone cream doesn't work to improve long-lasting postpartum depression, wait until you have finished nursing to try DHEA—and use it with the guidance of a health-care professional.

Breastfeeding Problems and Solutions

If you have never experienced any breastfeeding problems, you're one of the lucky ones. Almost every nursing mother has to deal with at least one breastfeeding-related issue, such as cracked nipples, engorgement, insufficient milk supply, mastitis, nipple pain, plugged ducts, and thrush. Unfortunately, many women abandon breastfeeding in the early weeks because of such problems. Fortunately, there are effective natural treatments that can usually overcome them. In this section, we will share the solutions that we have seen work best for nursing mothers.

CRACKED NIPPLES

If your nipple skin is delicate and your baby enjoys marathon nursing sessions, you may end up with this painful problem. Buy a tube of pure lanolin ointment—most stores that sell breastfeeding supplies carry it—and keep a thin coating of ointment on your nipples whenever your baby isn't nursing. The good thing about lanolin is that it will not harm your baby, so you don't need to wipe it off to nurse. Its texture actually can help the baby latch on properly.

To prevent cracked nipples, air them out frequently. If you would rather not go braless, turn the flaps of your nursing bra down for a while each day. Do not use plastic-lined breast shields; stick with washable cotton or disposables without plastic linings. Also try *Phytolacca decandra,* a homeopathic remedy, for cracked nipples. This remedy can also work well for mastitis.

ENGORGEMENT

This is most common in mothers in the early stages of nursing, soon after the milk first comes in. Your body and your baby are in the process of establishing their supply-and-demand relationship, and if your milk supply is greater than your baby's demand, you can end up with extremely swollen, football-hard breasts that hurt you and frustrate your baby's attempts to latch on.

Deal with engorgement promptly to avoid mastitis. Expressing some milk with a pump or by hand before feeding will make latch-on easier. According to breastfeeding expert Jack Newman, M.D., cabbage leaves are an excellent treatment for engorgement and breast inflammations. Place a cool raw leaf in each side of your nursing bra and change them often. (If your breasts aren't shaped like cabbages, roll the leaves with a rolling pin to make them more accommodating to your unique shape.)

INSUFFICIENT MILK SUPPLY

Many new mothers worry about low milk flow, but few actually have insufficient milk for their babies. As long as your baby is soiling and wetting diapers and seems contented after a feeding, your milk is flowing just fine. If you do need to augment your milk production, stopping the use of prescription or over-the-counter medicines may take care of the problem. The following are some other techniques for increasing your milk production:

- First and foremost, drink more water. If you aren't drinking enough, your milk production will go down.
- Nurse as often as possible. Eliminate all breast substitutes for your baby, including pacifiers and bottles. If your baby only gets the real thing, the constant stimulation will greatly increase your milk supply.

- Try switch feeding. Start nursing on one breast, and switch your baby over to the other breast five minutes later. Continue to switch back and forth every five minutes until the feeding ends.
- If your baby is already eating solids, decrease them for a day or two so that he will want to nurse more.
- Take a powdered calcium and magnesium supplement at night. This can improve milk flow and help you sleep better at night.
- Try using herbs. A wide variety of herbs work to increase milk production. Try goat rue, blessed thistle, milk thistle, nettles, alfalfa, red clover, hops, astragalus, thyme, or dill.
- Increase your consumption of green, leafy vegetables, which help to augment milk flow. If these don't agree with your baby, try adding liquid chlorophyll to your drinking water.
- Try the traditional European method for improving milk flow: Drink a dark beer! (Just one.)

MASTITIS

If breast inflammation is accompanied by flulike symptoms and intense pain, you probably have mastitis, an infection of breast tissue. The most important thing to do for this condition is rest. If you do not care for yourself properly during a bout of mastitis, you could end up with an abscess that requires lancing and draining.

Go directly to bed and nurse your baby as much as possible. If you can, enlist a friend or family member to help with your baby whenever you aren't nursing. Keep moist heat on the affected breast. Bundle up and let the fever run its course rather than lowering it artificially with a drug such as acetaminophen (Tylenol). Fever is your body's way of activating the immune system against the infection. The exception to this is a fever over 103°F, which should be brought down as quickly as possible. An enema of slightly cool water will often reduce a high fever, as will inducing diarrhea by taking buffered vitamin C powder in water (start by taking 1,000 milligrams of vitamin C dissolved in an 8-ounce glass of water, give it a few hours, then take gradually increased doses, up to as much as 5,000 milligrams, as needed). For the usual, low-grade fever (99°F to 102°F), rest, drink plenty of fluids, and take immunity-stimulating vitamins and herbs such as echinacea, olive leaf, vitamin C, and, once daily, about 5,000 international units of vitamin A.

If, after twenty-four hours of total rest and self-care, your symptoms are the same or worse, you may need to take antibiotics. Consult with your doctor. With or without antibiotics, mastitis usually takes two to five days to clear up completely.

NIPPLE PAIN

We hate to think of how many mothers give up on nursing because of this problem. The most important way to avoid nipple pain is to be sure your baby is latched on properly. With a newborn, it is almost never as simple as popping the baby on the breast and letting nature take its course. Once milk really begins to flow, two or three days postpartum, proper latching on can seem elusive. You may find you need to be surrounded by stacks of pillows, and even then you might wish you had a third hand to help you maintain the right positioning. If nursing hurts, even a little bit, consult with a lactation specialist for assistance.

Nipple pain that doesn't go away with proper positioning could be due to a breast infection or thrush.

PLUGGED DUCTS

A plugged duct is your body's early warning sign that you are pushing yourself too hard. Slow down and take the time to clear the duct out to avoid ending up with an infection. The plug feels like a hard lump, and there may be some engorgement or pain. Nurse from that side, massaging the breast while baby drinks, to try to loosen the plug. Massage from the armpits downward and toward the center of the breast. If you can, point baby's chin in the direction of the blockage. For example, use the football hold (cradling the baby under your arm) if the plug is in the lower outside quadrant of your breast. If the plug is on the armpit side of your breast, you can also try lying on your side next to your baby with the affected breast above him, and nurse him by dropping that breast down across the other one to his mouth. When the baby is done, pump off or hand-express any excess milk.

If you see a small blister on the nipple of the breast with the plugged duct, Dr. Jack Newman recommends opening it with a needle that has been sterilized by being held in a match's flame for a few seconds, then allowed to cool. This may allow you to gently squeeze out the blockage. Smooth an antibiotic ointment on the nipple to protect against infection (wipe the ointment off before nursing and reapply it afterward). For the plugged duct that won't let go, therapeutic ultrasound may do the trick. Ask your OB/GYN about this if necessary.

Dr. Newman suggests that women with recurrent plugged ducts take 1,200 milligrams of lecithin (a supplement usually made from soybeans) three to four times daily. Marshmallow—the herb, not the puffy, white, sugary snack you set aflame over campfires as a child—also can help clear up breast blockages and inflammations. Follow the dosage directions on the product label.

THRUSH

This sometimes itchy, sometimes painful condition is the result of the overgrowth of a yeast called *Candida albicans,* the same yeast that causes vaginal and intestinal yeast infections. You may develop an itchy rash on your nipple or experience pain when your baby nurses. If your baby's mouth is lined with white patches that don't wipe away easily, she has thrush, and you may have it too, even if you are not having symptoms. Thrush can also cause your baby to develop persistent diaper rash. The use of antibiotics is often the cause of yeast overgrowth because these drugs kill off "good bacteria" that normally keep yeasts in check.

While thrush is usually not dangerous, it can be uncomfortable. Nipple pain caused by thrush tends to last for a period after baby nurses, and may burn and radiate deeply into the breast. If there is no discomfort, however, you can just let thrush resolve on its own.

The best treatment is to repopulate those good bacteria with an acidophilus/bifidus supplement. Organic plain yogurt contains these bacteria and can be a good topical remedy for nipples. Your baby can take baby acidophilus powder in breast milk or directly from your nipples. The infection should clear up in a few days.

Birth Control While Breastfeeding

Many women who relied on oral contraceptives before starting a family feel at a loss when it comes time to think about birth control again. We believe that oral and injectable hormonal contraceptives should absolutely not be used by nursing mothers. The estrogens contained in oral contraceptives can dramatically diminish the quality and quantity of a mother's milk. We recommend against other hormonal forms of contraception as well. While low-estrogen hormonal contraceptives (such as progestin-only pills, implants such as Norplant, and injectable contraceptives such as Depo-Provera) do not have the same effect on milk supply as those containing estrogen, they can have adverse effects on your mood, and we do not know enough about what the progestins may do to the baby. We generally advise against the use of hormonal contraceptives in any case. They block your body's natural production of progesterone and can increase your lifetime risk of developing breast cancer.

What forms of contraception can work in harmony with nursing? In the first six months, mothers who breastfeed exclusively and on demand— no nipple substitutes, no bottles—are highly unlikely to become fertile again. However, if you are absolutely against becoming pregnant again so soon, use a barrier method of contraception such as a condom, diaphram, or cervical cap whenever you have intercourse, just to be safe. Of course, if you are not exclusively demand-feeding your baby, you could become fertile much sooner. Choose a nonhormonal method such as the intrauterine device (IUD), condoms, diaphragm, spermicide, or cervical cap.

Once your menstrual cycle returns and becomes regular, you can begin to track your fertile periods. The rhythm method does work very effectively if you carefully track your monthly ovulation, using body temperature and vaginal mucus to identify the time of ovulation, and use contraception or abstain during the fertile period that follows. This is the most natural way to avoid pregnancy and puts you in greater touch with your fertility. Dr. John Lee recommends the use of a small, lipstick-sized microscope called an Ovu-Tech that allows you to view your saliva. Specific changes in the saliva help you to know when you are fertile.

Maybe you are feeling, "I'd rather abstain, thank you very much." Many women complain of lack of sex drive postpartum. Very low progesterone and estrogen levels during the breastfeeding period can cause vaginal dryness that makes intercourse painful. After long days of baby care, some women feel "touched out" and do not want more physical closeness, even with their spouses. This can cause a partner to feel hurt and rejected, and resulting disagreements over sex can create unpleasant rifts at a time when you genuinely need each other's support. The most important thing to do is keep the lines of communication open. Talk to one another about your feelings and wishes. Keep in mind that if your libido is low, your body is telling you it's not the right time for intercourse. You and your mate might try to find some other way to express your love for each other.

Many women feel stressed out by their partners' pressure on them to have intercourse when it is literally the last thing on their own priority list—at least a few notches below ten more minutes of sleep. Do not be afraid to stand up for yourself on this one. It is easy to underestimate the added burden that this kind of spousal pressure creates on an already harried nursing mother. If this is a constant source of conflict, consider seeing a counselor together so that you can reach an agreement that works for both of you. For most women, libido returns naturally within a year after giving birth, and usually to some extent within about six months. Having your hormone levels checked, and using supplemental progesterone if necessary, may bring back your libido sooner.

Although there are many pharmaceutical drugs that should not be used while breastfeeding, there are some natural remedies, including herbs, that can be effective and safe for both you and your baby. In the next chapter, we will introduce you to some of our favorite natural remedies.

11

Using Herbs to Restore and Maintain Postpartum Health

Herbal medicine is thousands of years old, but only in the past few decades has it entered the realm of ultra-modern science. Herbs were mainstream medicine up until the advent of modern pharmaceuticals halfway through the twentieth century. At that point, drug companies figured out how to molecularly "tweak" plants, to refine them down to very specific active ingredients that would have much more targeted effects on the body than whole plants as they come from nature. Pharmaceuticals proved to be highly effective at making symptoms disappear and helping patients to feel better—fast.

Today, pharmaceutical drugs can offer near-instant relief from unpleasant symptoms of disease. Pain medicines wipe out headaches and menstrual cramps, cough syrup suppresses a nagging cough, antianxiety drugs soothe nervous feelings, and antihistamines control hay fever symptoms.

There is a darker side, however, to the bright picture of a world free of nagging symptoms. That includes the fact that a pregnant woman or nursing mother cannot pop any old pill whenever she feels like it because many pharmaceutical medications can harm her baby. Dangers exist for her, too—interactions between and side effects from prescription and over-the-counter drugs can hurt or even kill you. Our goal in writing this book has been to help you gain the kind of balance in your body and in your life that will make it unnecessary for you to use any more than the very occasional pharmaceutical drug.

Conventional Western, or allopathic, medicine works well to control symptoms—so well that we have become stuck in the mind-set that drugs are the only real way to deal with disease states. In the allopathic medical model, you wait until you get sick, and then you take a drug or drugs to relieve the symptoms so that you can get relief from your discomfort and get on with your life. In many cases, turning off the symptoms can be akin to turning off a fire alarm and failing to look for the reason the alarm sounded off in the first place.

Even when herbal medicine enters the conversation, most often it is in terms of the *treatment* of certain conditions. For instance, you have probably read about using echinacea to *treat* a cold, or black cohosh to *treat* uncomfortable menopausal symptoms. While it is true that these herbs can be effective for these problems, they work in a different way than pharmaceuticals work. Herbs don't work as "magic bullets," as many pharmaceuticals are purported to do. Instead, they tend to work to support the body's natural healing tendencies. The effects of herbs on the body are milder and more comprehensive than those of pharmaceuticals.

A person with any of a variety of vague complaints who goes to a conventional doctor is likely to walk out with a prescription to treat each complaint separately, while an herbalist would look for the big picture those symptoms paint and can design an herbal remedy to help the body ease itself back toward a state of balance. It follows that you should not expect immediate or strikingly obvious results from herbs, although this can sometimes occur. It is more likely, though, that you will notice a difference over time, and it may take weeks of diligent use before you feel them working.

Modern scientific research has shown us that herbs are effective medicine. After all, many prescription drugs are originally extracted from plants, or began their medicinal history as plant extracts that were then modified into patentable medicines not found in nature (medicines that are found in nature cannot be patented). We understand a great deal about how the active constituents work in the body; modern science studies those constituents carefully in hopes of deriving new drugs from them.

In this chapter, we will cover in detail only a few selected herbs that we feel offer great benefit for women who are in the process of pregnancy recovery. Little is known about interactions between herbs, and definitive scientific information on the safety of herbs for breastfeeding women is scant at best. Most herbs sold in stores advise pregnant and nursing women not to take them, but this is really because manufacturers are playing it safe in case of litigation. Pregnant and nursing women have used herbs for much longer than they have used drugs!

We have limited our discussion here to herbs with excellent safety profiles that can be used either separately or together by nursing mothers. If you are using any prescription drug on a regular basis, talk to your doctor or pharmacist about potential interactions between herbs and the drug. We focus first on adaptogenic herbs, which are herbs that offer general support to enhance the body's resilience in the face of stress. We have found that adaptogenic herbs can provide enormous benefits during the postpartum phase. We also discuss herbal antibiotics (unlike prescription antibiotics, these are herbs that help the body to fight off infection naturally); herbs for anxiety, coughs, and pain; and galactagogues, or herbs that support breast milk production.

Keep in mind that while the herbs recommended in this book are overwhelmingly safe when used properly, they should nevertheless be used under the supervision of a licensed health-care practitioner.

Adaptogenic Herbs

The whole concept of adaptogenic herbs is foreign to most practitioners and patients of Western medicine. These herbs are not used to cure a specific symptom or disease. Instead, they are used to restore the body's general natural balance. Adaptogens improve overall resistance to stress by supporting all of the body's systems, especially the immune system.

In traditional Chinese medicine (TCM), herbs that bring the body to a normalized, balanced place are referred to as *constitutionals*. Adaptogens actually go a little further than that by giving the body the ability to better withstand stress. Indigenous people who live in stressful environments almost always find a native adaptogenic herb that they use to help deal with the effects of stress.

SIBERIAN GINSENG

A Soviet scientist named I.I. Brekhman was responsible for the scientific research that brought ancient adaptogenic herbs into the twentieth century. He traveled to Siberia and asked people how they got through the long, bone-chilling winters. They told him about a plant that is known today as Siberian ginseng. His study of this herb led Dr. Brekhman to coin the term *adaptogen* to describe a whole class of herbs.

Researchers studied the herb's effects on some 40,000 factory workers, and found that regular use of Siberian ginseng improved productivity and stamina. Later, the studies expanded to include the Soviet Olympic team and the Soviet astronauts. From study to study, the effects were very consistent. Further research showed that adaptogens work better the longer you take them. It follows that they don't have an immediately noticeable effect, as a stimulant or a prescription drug would have.

It is not entirely clear yet exactly how adaptogens work. They seem to enhance endocrine function, preventing glands from producing either too much or too little of whatever they produce, such as estrogen, insulin, or thyroid hormone. In a postpartum situation, both blood sugar extremes— hypoglycemia (low blood sugar) and hyperglycemia (high blood sugar)— often strike, and Siberian ginseng seems to help balance either one of these conditions by affecting the way the body stores and releases sugar into the bloodstream. Adaptogenic herbs can also have beneficial effects on blood pressure.

Siberian ginseng seems to have a positive impact on immune function. Several studies have shown that when people who are undergoing chemotherapy or radiation for cancer take it, their immune systems better withstand the treatments.

Improvements in mental clarity and focus have been observed in studies of Siberian ginseng. One of the most common complaints we hear from women in the first months to years postpartum is that they often feel foggy or confused, and that they don't remember things as well as they used to. While some of this might be due to a lack of sleep, imbalanced hormones, or to the incredible amount of multitasking that is required of a new mom, there are probably biochemical reasons for this that we do not yet understand. The evidence is strong that Siberian ginseng can be a good choice for women with this complaint.

You are not likely to experience an immediate response to Siberian ginseng if you start taking it for fatigue, but if you take it over a period of weeks to months, you will notice that you have more energy and that your energy levels are sustained throughout the day. Your wounds will heal more quickly, your blood sugar will be more stable, and you will sleep better at night. The alertness brought about by this herb is not followed by the resounding crash characteristic of stimulants such as caffeine, ephedra, or guarana. A nursing mother can take Siberian ginseng without any concerns about stimulant effects on her baby.

Keep in mind that, botanically speaking, Siberian ginseng is not really ginseng. The true ginsengs, such as *Panax ginseng* (also called Asian ginseng), have been used in Asian medicine for thousands of years. The actual botanical name of Siberian ginseng is *Eleutherococcus senticosus,* and it is a member of an entirely different plant family than the true ginsengs, but it has many of the same properties when used medicinally. Siberian ginseng's common name is more descriptive of the herb's properties than its botanical origins.

According to Dr. Brekhman's research, and our clinical experience, Siberian ginseng is generally much better tolerated than Asian ginseng. Although the research on this is unclear, there is some evidence that Asian ginseng could have masculinizing effects in women. Siberian ginseng does not have any kind of masculinizing effect or any kind of effect on hormone balance that might be detrimental to women.

A good dosage of ginseng is about 300 milligrams in the morning and evening. Or follow the instructions on the product label.

SCHIZANDRA

For thousands of years, schizandra (*Schizandra chinensis,* also known as *wu wei zi*) has been used by Chinese women as a youth tonic and sexual rejuvenator. It has mild sedative effects, but also has adaptogenic effects similar to those of Siberian ginseng: it improves physical stamina and alertness, and staves off fatigue. Some herbalists recommend its use in the treatment of depression.

Unfortunately, research on many Chinese herbs is hard to find. They are rarely used alone, but are typically prescribed as part of a formula that contains five to ten other herbs. We do know that schizandra is traditionally used for all kinds of women's problems. It appears to support the detoxification processes of the liver, raising glutathione levels and helping the body to get rid of xenoestrogens and other hormone-disrupting chemicals.

Schizandra is safe and has been used by women since antiquity. You can most likely benefit from its adaptogenic properties without concern even if you are breastfeeding, and you may be able to use it for extended periods. However, since herbs are powerful medicine, we strongly recommend that you use herbs only under the guidance of a licensed practitioner who has experience with clinical herbology and can make dosage recommendations according to your body weight.

LICORICE

Americans think of licorice as a flavoring for candy. Actually, most versions of licorice candy don't have a single speck of licorice in them. Anise is the plant that gives American licorice candy its distinctive taste and smell. When licorice candy was first made, however, the herb licorice was added because of the sweetness of a compound called *glycyrrhizic acid* that it contains. Licorice (*Glycyrrhiza glabra*) is one of the best known and most useful medicinal herbs on the planet. It holds a place in the list of the top five herbs prescribed by practitioners of Chinese medicine—and for good reason.

Licorice has some adaptogenic properties. Specifically, it seems to help boost low blood pressure. In the West, herbs that raise blood pressure are considered to be dangerous. Information on herbs put out by the American Medical Association warns against licorice because of this effect, but we have found that in women with chronic fatigue, a mild blood pressure boost is exactly what is needed. Many women in the postpartum phase—especially in the first six weeks, when blood volume is still being built back up—complain of lightheadedness when they stand from a seated or lying-down position, and this is usually due to a strong dip in blood pressure. Using the herb licorice can help to alleviate this problem. Of course, if you have high blood pressure, or if you had pregnancy-induced hypertension or preeclampsia, you should avoid licorice. (You can still use deglycyrrhizinated licorice, or DGL, as recommended in Chapter 8, to help relieve heartburn and acid reflux.)

Licorice works as an antiviral agent, and helps your immune system to fight off a wide range of viruses and bacteria. Research has shown that women are more vulnerable to infections of all kinds during the first six months postpartum, and licorice—in addition to other immunity-boosting and antibiotic herbs, which we will discuss later in this chapter—is a wonderful herb to use during those months. Licorice is also soothing to mucous membranes throughout the body, which makes it ideal for the relief of uncomfortably inflamed nasal passages or lungs.

Finally, licorice has phytoestrogenic effects. These plant chemicals are not estrogens *per se*, but they do bind to some of the same receptors that estrogens bind to. The action of phytoestrogens can gently enhance or balance estrogen receptor activity, thus normalizing your body's ability to respond to estrogen during the hormonal peaks and valleys of the postpartum phase.

We recommend that women who use licorice take between 1,000 and 2,000 milligrams (1 and 2 grams) of the powdered root per day. There is some variation in the amount of active ingredient present in products of different herb manufacturers, and this can cause confusion when it comes to dosing. We recommend using a 10-to-1 concentrate, which means that ten pounds of licorice root were used to make one pound of the concentrate. The resulting herbal supplement is ten times more concentrated than a product that is basically ground-up root. Just a ¼ to ½ teaspoon of the concentrate is equivalent to 2,000 milligrams of straight ground licorice root. Whatever type of licorice extract you choose, there should be dosing instructions on the product label. Start at the low end of the dosage spectrum.

If you begin to retain fluid or experience a significant rise in blood pressure, you may be taking too much licorice root. Back off on the dose slightly to enjoy the beneficial effects without these problems.

Once again it is our strong recommendation that herbs be taken only under the guidance of a licensed practitioner who has clinical experience in this arena.

Antibiotic and Antiviral Herbs

Imagine this: In the midst of caring for your newborn, you are struck by a bad cold or bronchitis. Your doctor tells you that you can take over-the-counter medicines for your symptoms, and may prescribe antibiotics if he or she deems them necessary. You know from having read Chapter 10 of this book—and you know in your gut as well—that you really shouldn't use these medicines while nursing unless you absolutely need to. Fortunately, there are effective herbal alternatives to over-the-counter and prescription medications that can be used safely by a breastfeeding mother. These herbs are also useful for breast infections.

ASTRAGALUS

Astragalus (*Astragalus membranaceus*) has been used in TCM for thousands of years. It offers broad-spectrum support for the body's defenses against disease, but is especially effective against colds and flu. It can be used either on an ongoing basis as an immune tonic or short-term during an illness. Astragalus can also be given to children in low doses, and getting some through your milk will help keep your baby healthy. Use 1,000 to 2,000 milligrams a day (1 to 4 dropperfuls of tincture). An extra bonus if you need it: Astragalus also works to increase milk production.

ECHINACEA

Echinacea (*Echinacea angustifolia* and *Echinacea purpurea*) is a member of the daisy family. It was once relied upon by the American Great Plains Indians for the treatment of colds, coughs, sore throats, and a variety of other ills. A large body of research supports its use to enhance immune function during illness. In Germany, echinacea is a government-approved medicine for flu and chronic infections.

The popular notion that using echinacea over the long term can prevent illness is not supported by the research. In fact, there is some evidence that using it too often can actually decrease its effectiveness when you really need it. To treat any type of bacterial, viral, or fungal infection, take 500 to 4,000 milligrams per day of a product that contains a combination of *E. angustifolia* and *E. purpurea*. Start taking it at the first sign of illness and continue for seven to fourteen days. Divide the doses up as much as possible; take part of the dose in the morning and part in the evening, or some with each meal. Some people are allergic to echinacea. If taking it causes a worsening of symptoms such as congestion, stop taking it.

GARLIC

Garlic is an important antibiotic and antiviral herb. It is especially good for colds, flu, recurrent bowel complaints, stomach viruses, and yeast overgrowth. The research on garlic overwhelmingly supports its use as an antimicrobial, and because of its known anticancer effects, it makes sense to take supplemental garlic regularly.

To supplement with fresh garlic, peel one garlic clove (not the whole bulb, just a single clove!) and crush it with the flat side of a knife. Wait ten minutes for the enzymes in the garlic to completely activate its healing properties, then mix it with some honey and eat it. If chewing on this surprisingly tasty mixture seems a bit much, swallow the crushed clove with some water. If you get stomach pain or do not tolerate the taste and smell of garlic well, or if it doesn't seem to agree with your breastfeeding baby, try taking 300 to 900 milligrams of dried garlic extract daily. Avoid eating raw garlic on an empty stomach.

OLIVE LEAF

Olive leaf extract is one of our favorite immune-boosting herbs. Since the early nineteenth century, it has been used as a medicine for colds, flu, respiratory infections, and ear infections. It works quickly and safely to inhibit the growth of a whole menagerie of microbes. It is especially useful for people with chronic gastrointestinal troubles and for those who live or work in an environment where contagious diseases are often passed around. Use 500 to 3,000 milligrams per day. You can use olive leaf extract short term for acute disorders, or take it on an ongoing basis for chronic problems or to boost immunity.

Other Useful Herbs for Nursing Mothers

You can use herbs to replace pharmaceutical expectorants, painkillers, and sedatives. Their actions are not as dramatic or rapid as those of drugs, but, taken as directed, they can be very effective treatments that do not come with the risk of drug side effects. There are also several herbs that are useful for enhancing milk production. All are safe for nursing mothers if used according to the directions on the bottle or package. We will give you only the bare basics on these herbs. (For more thorough information on the use of medicinal herbs for you and your children, refer to *Smart Medicine for a Healthier Child* by Janet Zand, Bob Rountree, and Rachel Walton [Avery Publishing Group, 1994].)

EXPECTORANT HERBS

Expectorants assist the body in its efforts to expel mucus from the throat and lungs. A productive cough is your body's way of cleansing itself of toxic substances that are both causing and produced by respiratory illness. Taking a cough suppressant prevents this process and can actually prolong illness or make it worse. Try herbal expectorants such as wild cherry bark or anise. Herbalist Michael Tierra recommends that you inhale steam from water boiled with bay leaves, eucalyptus, and sage to help clear up lung congestion.

GALACTAGOGUE HERBS

Herbs that stimulate milk production are known as *galactagogues*. You can find them separately or in combinations in health food stores. Herbs in this category include blessed thistle, borage leaves (use this herb judiciously and with the help of an herbalist), fennel, goat's rue, milk thistle, nettles, raspberry leaf, and red clover.

SEDATIVE HERBS

Sedatives relax the muscles, decrease nervous tension, and help you to sleep more deeply. Try hops, chamomile, or passionflower, or a combination of these herbs. Chamomile is also an analgesic—it relieves pain by loosening painfully tightened muscles and by affecting the transmission of pain signals through the nervous system.

Herbs to Avoid

Just because herbs are natural, that does not mean that all herbs are safe under all circumstances—herbal medicines are medicines, after all. Some herbs have the effect of diminishing milk supply, and so obviously should not be used medicinally by nursing mothers. Herbs in this category include parsley (*Petroselinum crispum* or *P. sativum*) and sage (*Salvia officinalis*). Other herbs that should be *avoided* by nursing mothers include:

- Aloe (*Aloe vera*), taken internally (topical use is fine).
- Basil (*Ocimum basilicum*), in therapeutic doses (using it in cooking is fine).
- Black cohosh (*Cimicifuga racemosa*).
- Bladderwrack (*Fucus vesiculosus*).
- Bugleweed (*Ajuga reptans*).
- Cascara sagrada (*Frangula purshiana* or *Rhamnus purshiana*), an herb found in many stimulant laxatives.

- Coltsfoot (*Tussilago farfara*).
- Comfrey (*Symphytum officinale*), taken internally (topical use is fine).
- Elecampane (*Inula helenium*).
- Ephedra (*Ephedra* species, especially *E. sinica,* also known as *ma huang*).
- Fenugreek (*Trigonella foenum-graecum*).
- Foxglove (*Digitalis* species).
- Oregano (*Origanum vulgare*), in therapeutic doses (using it in cooking is fine).
- Periwinkle (*Vinca minor*).
- Senna (*Cassia* species).
- Sorrel (*Hibiscus sabdariffa*).
- Spearmint (*Mentha spicata*).
- Wormwood (*Artemisia absinthium*).

Herbs for Baby

Some herbs can be safe and effective remedies for colic, teething, general crankiness, and colds and other contagious bugs that strike little ones. Some of the most useful are:

- For colic or gas, chamomile, fennel (*not* fennel oil), and lemon balm.
- For teething: chamomile. Hyland's homeopathic teething tablets are also good.
- For colds and other infections, astragalus, echinacea, eyebright, goldenroot (*not* golden*seal*), and Oregon grape root.

For herbs to give your baby, you should be able to purchase glycerin herbal tinctures at your health food store. These tinctures are made with sugar rather than with alcohol. They taste good to babies and the small amount of sugar they contain is not harmful. Give them to your baby with an eyedropper or smear some on your nipple before he latches on. You can also brew herbal teas to give to your baby in a bottle. Fill a tea ball with dried herb and let it steep in hot water for at least ten minutes. Make herbal teas fairly weak for baby. *Do not* add honey to a tea made for your baby; children under the age of one should *never* be given honey. If you are nursing, you can simply take the herb yourself and a small amount will be passed on to your baby in your milk.

Now that you have some new resources for healing in your medicine cabinet, let's move on to an entirely different but equally important topic: Exercise.

12

The ABCs of Exercise

Few would deny that the pregnant body is glorious to behold. While it doesn't exactly match the description of Western culture's ideal form, the curvaceous body of a visibly pregnant woman draws admiring glances and compliments from many. If a picture is worth a thousand words, the picture of a woman about to bear a child is worth all of the words that seek to describe the miracle of new life coming into the world.

After gradual swelling and softening over ten months' time, the suddenly changed appearance of your body postpartum can be a bit of a shock. For the first week postpartum, your belly is still as round as it was when you were five months pregnant. Once your uterus contracts more fully, that roundness may subside—or, if you are still carrying a few excess pounds, it might not. For the first time in months, you can look down and see your legs, and if you gained a lot of weight with your pregnancy, you may find that you don't like what you see. If you are nursing, you may find that your newly larger breasts are a pleasing counterpart to the rest of your rounder figure—or you may be uncomfortable with your suddenly bountiful bosom.

In the first weeks postpartum, as you rest up from the birth and get acquainted with the new arrival, you may begin to wonder: When can I start exercising to try to get rid of this extra weight I've gained? How hard can I exercise? What's safe and what's unsafe for my body right now? And when am I going to find the time to exercise?

A Sensible Attitude Toward Postpartum Fitness

Our weight-conscious culture often fails to discriminate between *fitness* and *thinness*. Being thin does not make you fit, and being heavier than society's ideal does not necessarily mean you are unhealthy. It is true that obese people are at increased risk for heart disease and diabetes, but this is because people who eat poorly and avoid exercise have a better chance of ending up fat than those who watch what they eat and exercise regularly. If you are living a healthy lifestyle—getting your exercise and eating well—you may not be thin, but most likely you are fit. This is especially true of new moms, whose bodies tend to hang on to at least some of their pregnancy fat gain until their babies are weaned from the breast.

Recently, a news program did a story on a highly successful model who was prized for her reedlike thinness. It turned out that she was so thin because she was battling cancer. The weight of most women on television programs and in fashion magazines is that of someone who is ill, not someone who is healthy. Pleasingly plump talk show host Oprah Winfrey, who runs marathons, is an excellent example of radiant good health and fitness in a body that does not fit society's definition of perfection. And most would agree that she is beautiful.

When you are fit, you are energetic, strong, able to resist stress and infection, and able to meet the normal demands of daily life without pain or undue fatigue. Whether your physique is rail thin and rock hard, soft and bountiful, or some combination of these, you can be fit.

Our culture gives the most approval to the women who bounce back fast after pregnancy: "I can't believe you just had a baby—you look so *slim!*" Or, "It's so great that you're back to working out every day so soon!" Rarely do you hear anyone say, "You're taking it easy and not worrying about losing weight? That's terrific!" When we talk to women about their issues with weight and fitness, we find that many of them simply need to be told that it is perfectly okay to be heavier and to exercise more moderately during the first year postpartum, and that they should not expect to regain their prepregnancy figures while their babies are young.

Please keep this in mind as you read through this chapter. The conventional wisdom is that it took you nine months to gain the weight, and it will take at least as long as that to lose it. Pushing the envelope will not only drain your body of the resources it needs to recover from pregnancy and nourish your baby, but it will also most probably be an exercise in futility (pun intended). You need to be patient. In the meantime, instead of focusing on becoming *thin,* focus on becoming *fit.*

The Benefits and Risks of Postpartum Exercise

Starting a moderate exercise program during the postpartum months is beneficial in many ways. Regular exercise improves immune function and increases the production of antioxidant substances in the body. It helps you to sleep better at night and feel more energetic during the day. A brisk walk does wonders for depression or anxiety. A bout of exercise helps to suppress your appetite for sweets and junk food and increases your appetite for natural, nourishing foods. Flexibility and muscular strength stave off uneven strain on the skeleton that can lead to pain and injury over time. If your muscles are strong and your joints supple, you are less likely to throw your back out or injure yourself in some other way as you lift, bend, twist, and maneuver through your day. And if you start easing into exercise in a balanced and educated manner during the first postpartum year, the transition into more strenuous exercise later—should you choose to make that transition—is sure to be much smoother.

While some exercise is a very good thing for a new mom, doing too much too soon can be harmful. This is especially true for women who are low on the adrenal hormone cortisol. When you exercise, your adrenal glands pump out cortisol to increase your heart rate and breathing rate, and to increase blood flow to your muscles. As explained in Chapter 9,

Marcie's Story

Marcie worked out every day when she was pregnant. She didn't have to work and had lots of time to exercise, get the nursery ready, and just enjoy being pregnant, so she took advantage of it. She had always been a workout maniac so it wasn't a big adjustment for her. Every day she would swim laps, speed-walk, or take an aerobics class. She had been afraid she would get fat during pregnancy and so felt proud of how she stayed in shape. She also watched what she ate very carefully. From the back, you couldn't even tell she was pregnant, even when she was at her due date.

Her son Joseph's birth was difficult. Marcie had a very long labor and it took three hours to push him out. Everyone had told her, "Oh, you're in such good shape, it'll be quick and easy," but the opposite turned out to be true. Then, the big shock came: there was fat on her stomach and hips, which she hadn't been able to see when she was all full of baby. She felt so fat and flabby, she couldn't stand it. Even though her doctor told her to wait six weeks before starting an exercise program again, Marcie started going on walks only three days after giving birth, and started back into aerobics class ten days postpartum. Everyone was so impressed with how fast she had bounced back, but they didn't know how awful she was feeling.

She soon started to bleed heavily and felt very tired, and the asthma she had had since childhood began to flare up pretty badly. She thought she could push through it. But at her two-weeks' appointment with the doctor, he read her the riot act for not taking it easy. Her episiotomy wasn't healing well. She was wheezy and anemic. She was not making enough milk for her son. Marcie realized she had to stop focusing on losing weight and start focusing on getting rest and enjoying these fleeting early weeks of her son's life. So she went out and bought some flowing, elegant "mommy clothes" that hid her problem areas and got a great haircut, and that helped her to feel better about her new look.

there is a significant drop in cortisol levels postpartum. Going out for a run two weeks after giving birth will draw on the tapped resources of your adrenals before they are ready, and this will knock your recovering body out of balance. If laboratory tests show that your cortisol levels are low, you should postpone all but the most mild exercise until those levels return to normal.

You may have enjoyed an increased degree of flexibility during pregnancy. Your joints will still be loose for the first few weeks postpartum, and loose ligaments mean greater risk of injury. Exercising too hard in those first weeks can also delay the healing of episiotomy and cesarean incisions. If you hemorrhaged after giving birth, you may be anemic, and you will need to build up your iron levels for a while before you're ready to exercise.

Unrelenting or recurring muscle or joint pain in the hips, legs, or back can be related to the skeletal strain of late pregnancy and birth. If you have this problem, you may need to visit a skilled chiropractor or osteopath, who can assess any skeletal imbalances and correct them.

Starting to Exercise Again

An important point to remember about exercising postpartum is that you should not start too soon. But how soon is too soon? There are conflicting opinions on this. Some experts recommend waiting six weeks to do any exercise at all, while others tell new mothers that they can start as soon as the day after they give birth. In some rare instances, women are truly well enough to get up and walk a short distance the day after giving birth. This is more likely to be true of women who have given birth a few times before, and whose bodies are used to the transition into postpartum. On the other end of the continuum are women who have had a complicated birth and difficult recovery. Such women may need a full six weeks of rest before moving their bodies in any kind of vigorous way. Most women, however, fall somewhere between these two extremes. We recommend that new mothers do nothing but rest and recover for a full two weeks postpartum.

THE FIRST TWO WEEKS

For the first couple of days, if at all possible, stay in bed with your baby, nursing as often as possible and getting up only to use the bathroom and to do herbal sitz baths. One woman we know absolutely *had* to have a shower only three or so hours after giving birth to her first baby, and hobbled into the bathroom alone while her husband and baby dozed. She sustained a good smack on the head when she fainted in the stall. If, during those first few hours, you feel a sponge bath just doesn't get you clean enough, take a shower with your partner—sit on a stool and let him wash you and rinse you off (a hose attachment for your shower helps a great deal with this, and is a good thing to have for bathing your baby).

After the first two days, ease into regular activity gradually. Don't think that after a little bed rest you should scour the house and cook a three-course meal while your baby sleeps. Many expectant families enlist the help of friends and family, setting up a schedule that allows others to help out by bringing home-cooked meals and helping with chores and the care of older children.

One exception to this guideline: You can start doing Kegel exercises as soon as the day after giving birth. Hopefully, your doctor instructed you in how to do these, and advised you to do them regularly during pregnancy. If you haven't been doing Kegels, here's the basic exercise: Contract the muscles in your vagina as though you were holding back the flow of urine, and hold them that way for ten seconds at a time. Then relax. Do this whenever you think to do so, building up to five sets of ten repetitions three to four times a day. Kegels help to keep blood flowing to your genital and perineal areas, encouraging your body to heal from tearing, swelling, or bruising. They help to tone and firm the muscles in the vagina, counteracting that feeling some women have that their insides are going to slide out of them through their vaginas after giving birth. Kegels also help to control the leaking of urine that affects some women postpartum.

In some cultures, it is common practice for women to bind their bellies after giving birth. While belly binding is not medically necessary, and may not do anything to improve your shape, some of our patients tell us that it does feel quite good to gather everything in tightly. Belly binding may even help to speed the knitting together of separated abdominal muscles (more about this later in this chapter).

Some sporting goods stores sell snug midriff wraps that close with Velcro. Many women's clothing stores now sell camisoles, tank tops, or tube tops made from stretchy combinations of cotton and Lycra. Before your baby is born, look around and see if you can find anything like this to keep handy postpartum. If you have already had your baby, send a friend or relative out to search for something that feels snug and secure and allows you to nurse and rest comfortably.

AFTER THE FIRST TWO WEEKS

Walking is a good first exercise for both you and your newborn. Put your baby in a stroller or carrier and start walking. Start with a trip around the block, and gradually increase the distance you stroll.

If you have a gym membership and you have someone who can care for your baby for a couple of hours, check into postpartum exercise classes or gentle yoga classes. At home, you can begin doing the strengthening and stretching exercises described in the following pages one to three times a day while your baby naps or spends time with Dad.

Once you start exercising, be alert for signs that you may be working too hard. Watch for increased lochia flow (bleeding) after exercise sessions, especially in the first month postpartum. This is your body telling you to cool it. Otherwise, just listen to your body's signals. If your vagina, perineum, or cesarean incision are not healing well, if your breasts are too full and sore for even your most supportive bra, if you need a nap more than you need exercise, or if you experience dizziness or extreme fatigue, stop and try again tomorrow or the next day. You do not have to do this quickly, and rushing it will not make much difference in the end.

During the first month postpartum, don't worry too much about stretching your lower body. Your ligaments are still stretchy from the effects of the hormone relaxin. Nursing and carrying a newborn can cause the muscles in your shoulders, neck, and back to tighten, however. Stretches can help to relieve that tightness.

Easy Push-Ups

Get down on your hands and knees. Lower your chest down to the floor and then bring it back up. Try doing one set of ten with your elbows pointing out (to work your chest muscles), and another set with your elbows coming into your waist (to work the muscles on the backs of your arms). Most of your body weight should be supported on your knees. After the first week, try doing two sets of each per session.

Shoulder Blade Squeeze

This exercise helps to prevent the tense shoulders and upper back that new mothers often experience. Stand with your feet hip-width apart or sit in a straight-backed chair. Squeeze your shoulder blades down and toward each other, then release. Do this ten to twenty times per session.

Head and Shoulder Lifts

Most women have a diastasis, or separation in their abdominal muscles, after giving birth that feels as though someone had unzipped their abs down the center from top to bottom. This separation can be closed up with the right abdominal strengthening exercises. Before you try any abdominal exercises, check to see how wide your separation is. You can do this during this exercise.

Lie on your back and cross your arms over your chest. Inhale and slowly lift your chin toward your chest and curl the tops of your shoulders up off of the floor. Imagine that you are pressing your abdominal muscles down toward your belly button. Inhale as you release back down. Start out with ten repetitions and work up to twenty per session.

To check your diastasis, reach down with one hand as you hold your chin and shoulders up. Hold your hand with the palm facing your face and find the gap just above your belly button. You may be able to fit three or four fingers into that gap. If you have a diastasis wider than three fingers, take special care to build up your abdominal strength slowly. Don't attempt to do "crunches" (in which you lift your entire upper back off of the floor) or other more strenuous ab work until the gap has closed to less than three fingers in width. Wrapping your arms around your waist and hugging the two edges of the gap together as you work your abs will help close the gap.

Pelvic Tilt

This is an excellent first postpartum abdominal strengthener. Lie on your back with your knees bent and feet flat on the floor or your lower legs resting on the seat of a chair. Feel the small gap between the curve in your lower spine and the floor. Inhale deeply, and as you exhale, use your abdominal muscles to gently press your lower spine down. Imagine that your tailbone is curling up and around toward your navel. Release as you inhale again. Start with ten repetitions and work up to twenty per session.

Against-the-Wall Stretch

Stand facing a wall, about an arm's length away from it. Clasp your hands and bend forward from your hips, placing your forearms against the wall. Keep your knees slightly bent and your elbows as close together as possible as you slide your forearms down the wall. You should end up bent at the hips at about a 90-degree angle. Allow your chest and head to sink toward the floor and breathe deeply.

Half Head Rolls

Sit or stand comfortably with your back against a wall. Drop your right ear toward your right shoulder, keeping both shoulders relaxed (don't bring the shoulder up to meet the ear). Then slowly allow your head to roll forward, chin to chest, to the left, and back to the center. Repeat this a few times to loosen your neck and upper back muscles.

Cat Back, Dog Back

On your hands and knees, make your back flat, like a tabletop. Inhale and arch your back up toward the ceiling, tucking your chin toward your chest and your tailbone between your legs (this is the "cat back" portion of the exercise). Exhale, returning to the flat, neutral spine. Inhale again as you arch your back the other way, looking up to the ceiling and pointing your tailbone up (the "dog back" portion). Return to flat back again as you exhale. Repeat this a few times. Your baby will probably enjoy lying face up beneath you as you do this stretch.

Upside-Down Chest Stretch

Stand with your feet wider apart than your hips but not so wide that it strains anything, toes pointing forward. Clasp your hands behind your back, elbows straight, and inhale slowly and deeply. As you exhale, slowly bend forward until your head is hanging down. Do this slowly to prevent dizziness. If this feels like too much stretching in your legs or low back, bend your knees. Let your arms sink toward the floor behind your head. Stay in that position for at least ten seconds and be sure to come out of it slowly. If you feel dizzy or lightheaded even if you do this stretch slowly, do it in a chair with your knees spread and your feet flat on the floor.

Hamstring Stretch

Tight hamstrings put extra pressure on the lower back muscles, so be sure to do this stretch often. Sit on the floor with one leg extended straight out. Bend the other knee, let it fall to the side, and tuck the foot of the bent leg into the thigh of the straightened one. Straighten your back as much as possible, then lean over the straightened leg, pointing your tailbone back behind you. Gaze out at the extended foot. The bend should be happening in the hip joint, not the lower back. Feel your lower back with your hand—it should feel straight and flat, not rounded. You may be able to lean forward only slightly. That's okay; the object is not to put your nose on your knee, but to stretch the muscles in the back of the thigh of the straightened leg. Reach for the leg and gently draw your torso down toward it. Hold this position for at least half a minute, then switch legs.

Supported Backbend

Stack two or three pillows on the floor or on your bed. Sit right up against the stack with your back facing it, with your legs outstretched, then gently lie back over the pillows so that your head is hanging over the edge. Allow your arms to relax into whatever position feels best—try letting them stay by your sides, cross them over your chest, spread them wide, or raise them over your head. Breathe deeply as you stay in this position for up to two minutes. To get out of the backbend, roll to one side and off the pillows.

Child's Pose

This yoga pose is excellent for releasing tension from the entire body during and after pregnancy. Sit with your legs folded beneath you, so that you are sitting on your heels with your knees parted. Fold your body forward so that your torso sinks toward the floor between your thighs. Gently rest your forehead on the floor. You can extend your arms overhead, out to the sides, or down toward your feet. If you like, you can relax forward onto a pillow. Remain there for as long as you like, breathing deeply to allow deep inhalations to expand your lower and upper back.

Older babies that are crawling and pulling themselves up on objects love it when their moms stretch on the floor. Their favorite food source, piece of furniture, comforter, and entertainment system suddenly takes on a new role—jungle gym!

FOUR TO SIX WEEKS POSTPARTUM AND BEYOND

After the first four to six weeks have passed, you will be feeling much stronger. Your uterus will have gone almost completely back to its pre-pregnancy dimensions, although it is not likely that you will fit into anything but your baggiest prepregnancy clothing. At this point, your body is almost certainly ready for more vigorous activity. Some women are raring to go by a month postpartum, and others need a full six weeks before they feel really ready to work up a sweat.

If you were highly fit before pregnancy and kept up with workouts during pregnancy, you probably will have no trouble getting back into that groove—and more power to you if that is your plan. Everyone has heard of some woman who did an hour of step aerobics days before she gave birth and who was back training for a marathon within a month postpartum. Feel free to say hooray for her, but don't feel compelled to live up to her example, especially if you were not super-fit before and during pregnancy. You will only end up sore and miserable and, perhaps, even injured. More is not better when it comes to exercise. The key to maintaining a successful exercise program is to find what works for your

Jeannie's Story

Before Jeannie got pregnant at age forty, she worried constantly about gaining weight. Both of her parents were heavy and she had always had to be careful about what she ate. She weighed herself every day and changed her diet if she gained even one pound. If she ate too much one day she did extra jogging to burn off more calories. She felt as if she had things well under control. Of course, as soon as she got pregnant she had to let go of all of that (Jeannie thinks that might have been part of the reason she waited so long to have a child).

She tried to prepare myself for the shock of being heavy after her son Brian's birth, but she was surprised at how awful it felt to her. She says she thought she would go absolutely mad with self-loathing if she didn't get the weight off right away. Jeannie's plan was to go back to work three months after the baby was born, and she wanted to be back in her power suits by then. Hard exercise and calorie-counting had worked for her before, and so as soon as she felt able she got back to jogging and weight lifting at the gym. The gym she attended offered free baby-sitting for up to two hours daily, so she could spend all of that time working out.

Doing all of that exercise felt pretty good, but it didn't have much effect on her waistline or on her legs and hips. Jeannie could feel herself getting fitter but the fat clung to her frame. She knew that she could not eat much less than she was eating because she had to make milk for her son, and she was already supplementing his feedings with formula because he was gaining weight so slowly

Jeannie's return to work came and went, and her old power suits stayed hanging in the back of her closet. She had to buy new pants and skirts to wear to work instead. She no longer had time to go to the gym for two hours a day. Instead, she tried to incorporate more activity into her day at work. She climbed the stairs instead of using the elevator, conducted lunch meetings with coworkers during walks through the park, and kept small hand weights in her office to use during phone conversations. Occasionally she would go to the gym and do a harder workout. Only then did the weight begin to come off, and she still felt good. She lost twenty or so pounds and plateaued at about fifteen pounds above her prepregnancy weight.

By the time her son was eleven months old, Jeannie decided that it was all right to be a size twelve instead of a size eight. The important thing was that she learned that her life would not come to an end if she wasn't thin. She says she had to realize that it is all right to be heavier in order to let most of the extra weight come off, and if the rest does come off, it will be wonderful, but it won't really change anything—she will just take out her old suits again.

individual body. For one woman, climbing sheer rock walls is just the thing, while another woman may thrive on a daily slow swim in a warm pool, and yet another feels best when she practices yoga a few times a week.

Not too long ago, fitness guidelines dictated that you needed thirty to sixty minutes' worth of aerobic exercise—the kind that gets your heart pumping faster than 100 beats per minute—three times a week or more to be truly fit. On top of that, the guidelines recommended strength training two to three times a week to strengthen bones and muscles. Who has time for all of that? Certainly not a new mother. Those guidelines caused a lot of people to throw up their hands and give up on working out altogether.

Researchers then began to show that even mild physical activity, such as housework, walking around town to run errands, or gardening could offer the same long-term health benefits as more intense exercise. The notion that physical activity had to be continuous to be effective went the way of the dinosaurs when studies found that a few five- to ten-minute spells of activity throughout the day are just as health-supporting. This is true for women in the postpartum months as well as for anyone else.

Expand your notion of what exercise is. Taking your baby for a walk in a carrier or stroller is a great way to stimulate or soothe the child and improve your own fitness. Try walking to run errands whenever possible, and don't worry about getting your heart rate up to any particular level— that will happen on its own. Carrying your baby will strengthen your muscles and joints, and as your baby grows, so will your strength.

You should incorporate aerobic activity into every day in some way. One day you might do housework on and off throughout the day, walking and lifting and bending for ten minutes at a time. (Backpack baby carriers are great for toting baby while doing housework or cooking.) Another day you might go to the pool for a thirty-minute swim. Walking around in the mall with your baby and a friend or chasing older children around in the park also qualifies as exercise. Even the most irascible baby can be soothed by being gently bounced and rocked to music. Put your favorite music on the stereo, cuddle your baby in your arms, sling, or front pack—and dance!

Of course, if you like to go to the gym and lift weights and hit the treadmill, there is no reason not to do so once those first four to six weeks have passed. Moderate aerobic exercise increases the body's core temperature and makes it easier to burn fat and keep your energy levels high. Aerobic exercise also helps to burn off stress hormones. Overdoing it by allowing your heart rate to stay too high for too long (anaerobic exercise) actually triggers your body to produce more stress hormones, so balance is the key. Take the number 180 and subtract your age. The resulting number is your maximum safe heart rate. I recommend *not* allowing your heart rate to go above that rate for at least three months postpartum. For example, if you are thirty-five, you would subtract 35 from 180 to get 145, and you should not allow your heart rate to exceed 145 beats per minute. If you are feeling fatigued, it would be better to subtract 10 from that number and, in the case of this example, stay within a range of 125 to 135 beats per minute for the three-month period after you give birth. Work back into your prepregnancy routine gradually, and do not expect your body to be transformed rapidly back to its former state. It really does take about nine months, no matter how hard you work at it—so why deplete your body and stress yourself out needlessly?

In the following sections, we describe some more strenuous exercises you can do to help strengthen your muscles and stabilize your joints, even as you continue doing the stretching exercises described earlier in this chapter. You can use these strengthening exercises in preparation for more vigorous activities, or simply stick with them over the long term to maintain strength and stability. Try to do them at least three times a week. For the last two exercises discussed, the Seated Rear Dumbbell Fly and the Seated Lat Row, you will need some light, handheld weights. Almost everyone has some of these collecting dust in some corner of the house.

Start with three- to five-pounders and work up to heavier ones. These exercises will help to balance the strain of carrying your baby all day. They work the muscles across your upper back and the latissimus dorsi muscles, which run from your lower spine up to your shoulders.

Kegels with Wall Sit

Starting at four to six weeks after the baby is born, if you like, you can try substituting this more difficult version of Kegel exercise for the gentler type described earlier.

Stand with your back against a wall, then step both feet away from the wall about eighteen inches. Slide your tailbone down the wall into a partial squat. This will feel quite intense in your thigh muscles; you may be able to go down only a few inches at first. Hold the partial squat and do fast Kegels, contracting and releasing one to two times per second for fifteen to thirty seconds. Then slide back up the wall, straightening your legs.

Turned-Out Squats with Baby

If you have ever studied ballet, you might remember this as second-position pliés. It is a terrific exercise for strengthening the pelvic floor muscles, inner thighs, and lower back.

Hold your baby firmly against you or put him in a front pack or sling. Stand tall and place your feet as far apart apart as you can comfortably, letting your toes turn out slightly. Bend your knees in the same direction your toes are pointing, actively rotating your thighs out and away from each other. You should feel some effort in the muscles along the back of your hips. Keep your torso straight up and down as you lower your pelvis toward the floor. Go as far as you can comfortably, then come back up, maintaining the outward rotation in your legs. If you can, hold a Kegel gently throughout the exercise. Repeat this five to ten times. If your balance is challenged during this exercise, hold on to a chair back with both hands.

Baby Overhead Press

You probably already do this countless times a day. Hold your baby at chest level and raise her above your head, straightening your arms, then lower her back down. Repeat this ten to twenty times. An optional addition to this exercise is cooing, making funny faces, and giggling with your "airborne" baby!

Leg Slide

This is an excellent abdominal strengthener. Lie on your back with your knees bent and your feet flat on the floor. Press your lower back onto the floor, drawing your belly button down toward your tailbone. Slide your feet away from your body, straightening your knees until you can no longer keep your lower back on the floor, then return your feet to the starting position. You can do this one with your baby sitting on your hips. Do ten to fifteen repetitions per session.

Double Crunch with Baby

Lie on your back on the floor with your baby lying face down on the shins of your bent legs. Hold on to baby and lift your entire upper back off the floor, bringing your knees toward your forehead as you lift your head and shoulders. This is a good chance to start counting for your baby! Go for fifteen to twenty repetitions. When you feel strong enough, add a second set.

Push-ups with Baby

You are probably strong enough now to do "girl push-ups," in which you straighten your body but rest on your knees rather than on your feet. Put your baby down between your hands and give him a kiss with each of your ten to twenty repetitions.

Seated Rear Dumbbell Fly

Hold a weight in each hand and sit in a chair. Plant both feet firmly on the floor and lean your torso forward, so that it rests on your thighs. Hold the weights with your palms facing each other. Keeping your elbows slightly bent, lift the weights up and out to the side, as though you were flapping your wings. Keep the motion smooth, slow, and regular. Repeat ten to fifteen times, and then rest, letting the weights pull your arms down in a stretch. Add a second set when you feel strong enough.

Seated Lat Row

Hold a weight in each hand and sit in a chair. Plant both feet firmly on the floor and lean your torso forward, so that it rests on your thighs. Pull your elbows back along your sides, letting the weights hang down toward the floor. Try to touch your elbows together behind your back. You won't be able to, but if you work in this way, you will be working the right muscles. Repeat ten to fifteen times, then rest. Add a second set when it feels easy.

Breastfeeding and Exercise

If you are nursing, you may have a new challenge on your hands when it comes time to do more vigorous exercise: breasts that are bigger and more sensitive to jarring and bouncing than they have ever been before. If you plan to do fast walking, jogging, or anything else that causes your breasts to bounce, it is a good idea to invest in a few supportive sports bras that minimize motion by pressing your breasts flat. Wear these bras for exercise only. The pressure they exert can lead to plugged ducts or mastitis if you wear them over longer periods. Also, nurse your baby before you work out. If you time it right, your hungry baby can empty your breasts and be ready for a nice long nap while you exercise.

Some women report that their babies do not like the taste of their milk right after a hard bout of exercise. Lactic acid that builds up during hard exertion can make breast milk bitter, but moderate exercise should not pose this problem. If it does, hand-express or pump off some milk before the postworkout feeding.

A Final Word about Exercise: Do What You Can

The exercises described in this chapter should be enough to move you toward increased fitness in the postpartum months. They are appropriate whether you have never worked out in your life or have been a sports-woman since you were in diapers yourself.

If you cannot stick to an exercise program after your baby is born, don't beat yourself up about it. Do what you can and add more when you feel able to. Every little bit you do helps your body move toward a fitter state. If, however, you are not exercising and find that you are feeling excessively tired or depressed, your body hurts, you are constantly getting sick, or you are gaining weight postpartum, keep in mind that exercise has healing effects on all of these symptoms. Remember that this isn't an all-or-nothing proposition, and let it be a natural part of your daily life.

13

A Healthier Outlook

There is no question that having a baby can be one of the most stressful events of a woman's life. Beyond the physical stresses, which we have discussed at length throughout this book, many mothers fall straight out of their post-childbirth convalescence onto the treadmill of "doing it all"— and pretending to like it. Many of the moms we have talked to and treated feel the strain of having to be a full-time parent, hold down a part-time or full-time job, and also shoulder the responsibilities of cooking and keeping house. "I know women are supposed to be able to multitask," said one busy single mother of two, "but this is ridiculous. I get it all done, but nothing gets done well, and by the end of the day I have zero time to take care of my own needs."

Let's face it: Our fast-paced culture places enormous emphasis on financial and professional success, on appearances and acquisition, and very little on creating an environment where pregnancy, childbearing, and mothering are highly valued and supported. Even if you follow the advice in this book to the letter, and your health is restored and you feel physically better than you have in years, the stresses you have to deal with each day are still going to be there every morning when you wake up. No amount of good nutrition is going to change that, although it is certainly easier to face those stresses if you are not feeling ill or depressed.

It could be argued that the type of medicine most commonly practiced in America today—what we have referred to throughout this book as *mainstream* or *conventional* medicine—is the only form of medicine that has ever completely disregarded the role of the mind, the spirit, and the emotions in maintenance of good health. While this attitude is slowly changing, there is still an overwhelming bias against the notion that the way you think has profound effects on the way your body feels and heals from disease, despite solid scientific evidence of this mind-body link. As practitioners of functional nutrition, chiropractic, and traditional Chinese medicine (TCM), we recognize that many of our patients need not only to change the way they eat, exercise, and otherwise nourish their bodies, but also to change the way they *think*.

One of the best scientific illustrations of the mind-body connection is the placebo effect. When ill people who think they're getting a medicine that will help them to heal are instead given an inert sugar pill, many of them *do* heal. On the other hand, people who think they are getting medicine may also exhibit side effects, especially if they are told which ones to expect. When a doctor tells a trusting and "compliant" patient that he or she has only a certain number of months to live, it often happens that the patient dies right on schedule. Some patients, however, are less trusting and compliant, and these are the patients who usually outlive their doctors' predictions.

Much research has been done on the links between the mental images we allow to form in our mind's eyes and the effects of these images on the nervous system and the immune system. In fact, a new branch of scientific research, known as *psychoneuroimmunology*, has been created to further our understanding of the ways in which imagining and thinking can affect brain and immune system function. Psychoneuroimmunological research clearly shows that in people who are often worried or stressed out, immunity is hampered enough to increase susceptibility to infection, autoimmune disease, and even cancer. Negative emotions literally prevent the organs and glands that make up the immune system from doing their jobs.

It is clear that certain people deal with stress better than others. Some people can perform brain surgery or open-heart surgery five days a week, or work sitting on a girder dozens of stories above the ground, while others can barely handle the stresses of much lower-risk professions. One patient told us about a woman who is something of a living legend in the town where they live: She has three sets of twin boys, all under the age of ten, plus an infant son, and yet she appears relaxed and not the least bit harried. In comparison, some women feel overwhelmed caring for a single child.

Many people cannot handle stresses that seem benign to others, and often these low-tolerance people end up with life-threatening addictions to substances that help them escape what they perceive to be unbearable stresses. Such differences make one woman much more successful than another at moving through the stress of having a baby, losing sleep, lacking adequate support from her partner (no matter how much support a new mother's partner gives, it rarely seems like enough), and generally running the gauntlet of pregnancy, birthing, and parenthood. Fortunately, there are specific practices that we know can help a woman to move in the direction of dealing with the stresses in her life more successfully. We will look at a few of these in this chapter.

Embracing a Spiritual Practice

Prayer, meditation, contemplation, and positive creative visualization have all been shown to support good immune function and good physical and psychological health in general. Inspirational reading or listening to meditation or relaxation tapes can be very soothing and replenishing. Yoga, tai chi, and chi kung are traditional meditative practices that help you to focus your energies and remember what is really important.

Using your creative imagination to feed your brain positive images helps to relax your nervous system, soothe your emotions, and stimulate your hormonal and immune systems to release healing substances into your bloodstream. The pineal gland, the seat of the creative imagination, is a way station that mediates the energy and images between the physical, emotional, mental, and spiritual bodies of a human being. For example, a

262 ■ A Natural Guide to Pregnancy and Postpartum Health

person can be driving a car in New York City while remembering feelings and thoughts generated by walking and talking with a friend in Paris years ago. The physical body is driving, while the emotional body is reliving the feelings or emotions generated by calling forth the images of that walk in Paris. Simultaneously, the mind is remembering and thinking about the ideas shared in that talk that took place many years ago, while the soul (the dispassionate observer) gleans the lesson in a nonjudgmental way. The images that we allow to enter our image-maker for embellishment have an effect on the functioning of the nervous, endocrine, and immune systems, and, therefore, on every other system in the body. Our attitudes and attention are the only aspects of our multidimensional being that we actually have any real control over. But this is profound—it is like having a hand on the rudder of a boat. We do not control the wind or the waves, but we can affect the direction of travel by means of the rudder. Similarly, the images you entertain profoundly affect the hypothalamus (sometimes called the emotional brain) and, consequently, the neural, hormonal, and immune-system chemicals our bodies produce. Don't go to sleep allowing troubling news images to negatively influence the chemicals your brain makes. Before going to bed, take a few minutes to find some peace, perspective, and solace. Read something uplifting. Recite a comforting prayer or poem. Give your image-maker positive, nourishing images to embellish. Find a way to feel and trust the love inside of you that is part of the great source of all life that lives within us.

We cannot recommend highly enough that you find a way to add one of these practices to your daily schedule. Spiritual practices quiet the body and mind, allowing them to settle back into their natural balance. When you sit quietly and focus on your breath, or pray to whatever higher power you believe in, you can allow the universe to take care of you rather than your taking care of anyone else. Spiritual practices allow you to step back from the dirty diapers, the spilled pea purée, and the other minutiae of motherhood to see the larger context within which those minutiae fit. Stepping back in this way and looking at the big picture can help you through the difficult times.

If you engage in some form of spiritual practice faithfully, you will find that the benefits spill over into your day-to-day activities. Rather than screaming at your toddler in frustration after he has pulled all of the freshly folded laundry out of the drawers, you might take a deep breath and relax into the mess.

Your spiritual practice is a time just for you. If you can, try to take ten to thirty minutes, once or twice a day, in a quiet space. Let your partner take care of the kids, out of earshot from where you are. If you are not sure what exactly to do once you have found this space, buy a book on meditation or attend a class for some guidance.

The Importance of Sleep

During your spiritual practice, you may find yourself nodding off. That is perfectly understandable, especially if you are not getting the sleep you need. In the United States, many people tend to think that sleep is irrelevant—that they should be able to chug along like the pink bunny on the battery commercials until they drop. The truth is that adequate sleep is healing and necessary, especially for a new mother. Sleep is something to look forward to, to relish, and to embrace, not something to be snatched whenever there is nothing pressing that needs to be done. We believe that a good night's sleep—and naps, when necessary—ought to be higher on everyone's priority list.

In our experience, the mothers who stay particularly healthy postpartum are the ones who allow themselves to sleep as much as they feel necessary. Most say that they took two- to three-hour naps every day for the first six months of their babies' lives. They didn't jump up to clean house or cook or pay bills when baby fell asleep. When their babies slept, they slept. Another perk: Those naps provided for bonding and snuggling time with their babies.

Being on the same sleep-wake cycle during the first months of the baby's life also helps to establish a trusting rapport between mother and child. Moms who go back to work within weeks of giving birth don't get the benefit of these daytime naps with their little ones, and their health can suffer as a result.

Certain types of brain waves—known as delta- and theta-waves—

that are generally accessed only in deep sleep trigger the brain to produce beneficial hormones like melatonin, growth hormone, dehydroepiandrosterone (DHEA), and sex hormones. Deep sleep also allows the brain to restore its supply of neurotransmitters that allow the cells of the nervous system to communicate with one another and with the rest of the systems of the body.

Instinctive Parenting

Every new mother has to cope with some unsolicited advice on how to parent—from her own parents, from well-meaning friends, even from strangers passing by on the street. Bookstores and libraries stock dozens of books that tell mothers how to keep their children happy, how to avoid spoiling them, how to get them to sleep through the night, how to encourage their intelligence and artistic abilities, and how to keep them healthy. We have heard more than one mother complain that there is too much information, much of it conflicting. With so much information and advice, it is hard to listen to one's instincts without some level of self-doubt.

What it all boils down to, however, is providing a good balance between the needs of the baby and the needs of the mother. If her baby is happy, appropriately stimulated, learning, and calm, a mother feels as though she's doing her job well. If her baby is fussy, bored, developmentally delayed, or prone to fits of screaming, the mother is stressed out and wonders what she is doing wrong.

We are not parenting experts, but we have noticed that women who practice a certain style of parenting, called *attachment parenting,* tend to have a somewhat easier and smoother time during the first few months postpartum. Attachment parenting involves two major guidelines. Neither guideline works for everyone, but if you find that either or both works for you, go ahead and put it to use. Whatever your approach, keep in mind that *you know best how to mother your own children,* and no book or theory can change that. Listen to your instincts, and if they tell you that these practices are right for you, great; if not, do what feels best and brings the greatest results and satisfaction.

The first and most important tenet of attachment parenting is that babies, before they are able to move around on their own, should be carried and held whenever possible. Most small babies do not want to be put down for any length of time, not even in a stroller or car seat, and put up a considerable fuss until they are picked up and held. Babies that are carried most of the time are calmer and cry less. As these children grow older, they tend to be less clingy, because their need for physical closeness to their caregivers has been fulfilled; they feel more secure when it comes time to explore the world. Rapport between mother and baby is improved tremendously when the baby is in near-constant physical contact with the mom. Other caregivers, including Dad, can take turns carrying and holding the baby when you need a break or if you must work.

To make this amount of carrying and holding your baby an easier proposition, invest in a few different baby carriers that allow you to tote your little one hands-free. Then you will be able to go about your daily life while baby observes and naps from his comfy perch. Your baby's brain and nervous system development are promoted by constant movement and observation of you at your everyday tasks. Most of the mothers we have talked with like front packs and over-the-shoulder slings. The advantage of the sling is that it is versatile and can be used, with a few minor adjustments, to nurse discreetly in public. If your baby falls asleep in the sling, you can simply take the sling off while she is in it and lay her down on a bed or in her crib. Pediatrician William Sears, M.D., one of the best known proponents of attachment parenting, calls this carrying period *babywearing*. Generally, it lasts from birth until the baby begins to crawl, walk, and engage in independent play—somewhere around nine months.

The second recommendation of attachment parenting is co-sleeping— sleeping with your baby. Modern American convention frowns upon this practice, citing the dangers of baby being squashed by sleeping parents or being at increased risk of sudden infant death syndrome (SIDS). There are recorded instances of intoxicated or grossly overweight parents harming their children while co-sleeping, but otherwise, it is a perfectly safe practice, and has not been shown to increase SIDS risk.

Many parents who put their babies down in cribs to sleep end up bringing their babies into their beds practically every night because it is easier than continually getting up to feed the baby and soothe her back to a deep enough sleep to slip her back into her crib.

In most cases, mothers who sleep with their infants during those first months sleep better. Such a mother does not have to get up for nighttime feedings, but can simply roll over and offer baby the breast as soon as she starts looking for it. The baby never gets to the point of panicked wailing, and so is more quickly soothed back to sleep. And co-sleeping mothers we know tell us that waking up with their babies is one of the most magical parts of their day. Mothers who have to return to work soon after giving birth benefit most from co-sleeping, which allows them time for bonding that they may miss out on during the day.

If you or your spouse have reservations about sharing your bed with your baby, you can try keeping baby's crib right next to your bed, or you can invest in a co-sleeper—a crib designed to attach to the side of the bed, creating a small extension where the baby can sleep within arm's reach. Of course, some parents and children don't sleep well together, and do better with the more typical parents-in-bed, baby-in-crib-in-nursery setup. Again—it's all about what works best for your family.

If you would like to know more about babywearing, co-sleeping, or other attachment parenting practices, refer to the excellent books on baby care by William Sears, M.D. Other excellent books that may make mothering easier are listed in the Resources section at the back of this book.

It has been our pleasure to offer you this natural guide to pregnancy and postpartum health. We passionately believe that the concept of pregnancy recovery—the utilization of diet, rest, and therapeutic dosages of essential nutrients to restore depleted nutritional reserves—is long overdue. Too many postpartum women have been given humiliating diagnoses and treatments for ills that could have been resolved nutritionally. As we have shown, all the metabolic pathways and processes of the body need essential nutrients to function optimally. It is far too easy to become deficient in these basic building blocks of life. Women who have given birth are particularly vulnerable to these deficiencies and pay a dear price in physical and emotional health when the need to replenish their bodies' nutritional reserves is ignored.

Our fondest hope is that mothers everywhere will understand and embrace the importance of participating in a natural program to restore their own nutritional and energetic reserves. If your present doctor scoffs at these ideas, find one who knows the importance of nutrition and what tests to run to help you. We look forward to a time when all doctors will be trained to know the nutritional needs of all the basic metabolic processes and help all postpartum women to restore their health naturally. In the meantime, there are already many doctors who have this knowledge and know how to run the lab tests that enable them to determine exactly which nutrients your body is deficient in. Seek them out. Some of these doctors are medical doctors, some are chiropractors, some are naturopaths, some are osteopaths, and some are acupuncturists. May you find those who genuinely know how to help. We wish you good health!

References

CHAPTER ONE: I HAVE A BEAUTIFUL BABY. WHY DO I FEEL SO TERRIBLE?

Breggin, Peter R., with Ginger Ross Breggin, *Talking Back to Prozac: What Doctors Won't Tell You About Today's Most Controversial Drug* (New York, NY: St. Martin's Press, 1994).

Buist, A., "Treating Mental Illness in Lactating Women," *Medscape Women's Health* 6(2) (March 2001): 3.

Byrd, J.E., et al., "Sexuality During Pregnancy and the Year Postpartum," *Journal of Family Practice* 47(4) (October 1998): 305–308.

Gjerdingen, D.K., "The Effects of Social Support on Women's Health During Pregnancy, Labor and Delivery, and the Postpartum Period," *Family Medicine* 23(5) (July 1991): 370–375.

Gjerdingen, D.K., and D. Froberg, "Predictors of Health in New Mothers," *Social Science and Medicine* 33(12) (1991):1399–1407.

Glazener, C.M., "Sexual Function after Childbirth: Women's Experiences, Persistent Morbidity and Lack of Professional Recognition," *British Journal of Obstetrics and Gynecology* 104(3) (March 1997): 330–335.

Glenmullen, Joseph, *Prozac Backlash* (New York, NY: Simon and Schuster, 2000).

Huysman, Arlene M., *A Mother's Tears: Understanding the Mood Swings that Follow Childbirth* (New York, NY: Seven Stories Press, 1998).

Hendrick, V., et al., "Fluoxetine and Norfluoxetine Concentrations in Nursing Infants and Breast Milk," *Biological Psychiatry* 50(10) (15 November 2001): 775–782.

Lester, B.M., et al., "Possible Association between Fluoxetine Hydrochloride and Colic in an Infant," *Journal of the American Academy of Child and Adolescent Psychiatry* 132(6) (November 1993): 1253–1255.

Newport, D.J., M.M. Wilcox, and Z.N. Stowe, "Antidepressants during Pregnancy and Lactation: Defining Exposure and Treatment Issues," *Seminars in Perinatology* 25(3) (June 2001): 177–190.

Yoshida, K., et al., "Fluoxetine in Breast-Milk and Developmental Outcome of Breast-Fed Infants," *British Journal of Psychiatry* 172 (February 1998): 175–178.

CHAPTER THREE: HOW NUTRIENT DEPLETION SETS
THE STAGE FOR POSTPARTUM AILMENTS

Bland, Jeffrey, *Clinical Nutrition: A Functional Approach* (Gig Harbor, WA: The Institute for Functional Medicine, Inc., 1998).

Braverman, Eric R., and Carl C. Pfeiffer, *The Healing Nutrients Within* (New Canaan, CT: Keats Publishing, 1987).

Cott, J., "Omega-3 Fatty Acids and Pregnancy," *Alternative Therapies in Women's Health* (12) (December 2000): 89–96.

Enig, Mary, *Know Your Fats* (Silver Spring, MD: Bethesda Press, 2000).

Murray, Michael, *Dr. Murray's Total Body Tune-Up* (New York, NY: Bantam Books, 2000).

Pelton, Ross, James B. LaValle, and Ernest B. Hawkins, *Drug-Induced Nutrient Depletion Handbook* (Hudson, OH: Lexi-Comp, 2000).

Pizzorno, Joseph, *Total Wellness* (Rocklin CA: Prima Publishing, 1998).

Schmidt, Michael A., *Smart Fats: How Dietary Fats and Oils Affect Mental, Physical, and Emotional Intelligence* (Berkeley CA: Frog, Ltd., 1997).

CHAPTER FIVE: BUILDING NUTRIENT
RESERVES WITH DIET

Butte, N.F., et al., "Adjustments in Energy Expenditure and Substrate Utilization during Late Pregnancy and Lactation," *American Journal of Clinical Nutrition* 69(2) (February 1999): 299–307.

Catalano P.M., "Pregnancy and Lactation in Relation to Range of Acceptable Carbohydrate and Fat Intake," *European Journal of Clinical Nutrition* 53 (April 1999) (Supplement 1): S124–131.

Cherian, G., and J.S. Sim, "Changes in the Breast Milk Fatty Acids and Plasma Lipids of Nursing Mothers Following Consumption of N-3 Polyunsaturated Fatty Acid Enriched Eggs," *Nutrition* 12(1) (January 1996): 8–12.

Fidler, N., et al., "Docosahexaenoic Acid Transfer into Human Milk after Dietary Supplementation: A Randomized Clinical Trial," *Journal of Lipid Research* 41(9) (September 2000): 1376–1383.

Naylor, K.E., et al., "The Effect of Pregnancy on Bone Density and Bone Turnover," *Journal of Bone Mineral Research* 15(1) (January 2000):129–137.

Scopesi, F., et al., "Maternal Dietary PUFAs Intake and Human Milk Content Relationships during the First Month of Lactation," *Clinical Nutrition* 20(5) (October 2001): 393–397.

Stoll, Andrew, *The Omega-3 Connection* (New York, NY: Simon & Schuster, 2001).

CHAPTER NINE: USING HORMONES
TO REGAIN BALANCE AFTER PREGNANCY

Abou-Saleh, M.T., et al., "Hormonal Aspects of Postpartum Depression," *Psychoneuroendocrinology* 23(5) (July 1998): 465–475.

Arem, Ridha, *The Thyroid Solution* (New York, NY: Ballantine Books, 1999).

Bell, A.W., and D.E. Baumann, "Adaptations of Glucose Metabolism during Pregnancy and Lactation," *Journal of Mammary Gland Biology and Neoplasia* 2(3) (July 1997): 265–278.

Bloch, M., et al., "Effects of Gonadal Steroids in Women with a History of Postpartum Depression," *American Journal of Psychiatry* 157(6) (June 2000): 924–930.

Buckwalter, J.G., et al., "Pregnancy, the Postpartum, and Steroid Hormones: Effects on Cognition and Mood," *Psychoneuroendocrinology* 124(1) (January 1999): 581.

Horst, R.L., J.P. Goff, and T.A. Reinhardt, "Calcium and Vitamin D Metabolism during Lactation," *Journal of Mammary Gland Biology and Neoplasia* 2(3) (July 1997): 253–263.

Kuhl, C., "Etiology and Pathogenesis of Gestational Diabetes," *Diabetes Care* 21 (August 1998) (Supplement 2): B19–26.

Lawrie, T.A., A. Herxheimer, and K. Dalton, "Oestrogens and Progestogens for Preventing and Treating Postnatal Depression," *Cochrane Database System Review* 2 (2000): CD001690.

Lee, John, Jesse Hanley, and Virginia Hopkins, *What Your Doctor May Not Tell You About Premenopause* (New York, NY: Warner Books, 2000).

Mastorakos, G., and I. Ilias, "Maternal Hypothalamic-Pituitary-Adrenal Axis in Pregnancy and the Postpartum Period. Postpartum-Related Disorders," *Annals of the New York Academy of Sciences* 900 (2000): 95–106.

Stagnaro-Green, A., "Autoimmune Thyroid Disease: Recognizing, Understanding, and Treating Postpartum Thyroiditis," *Endocrinology and Metabolism Clinics of North America* 29(2) (June 2000): 417–430.

Uvnas-Moberg, K., "Oxytocin May Mediate the Benefits of Positive Social Interaction and Emotions," *Psychoneuroendocrinology* 23(8) (November 1998): 819–835.

Wilder, R.L., "Hormones, Pregnancy, and Autoimmune Diseases," *Annals of the New York Academy of Sciences* 840 (1 May 1998): 45–50.

CHAPTER TEN: THE BREASTFEEDING FACTOR

La Leche League International, *The Womanly Art of Breastfeeding* (New York, NY: Penguin Books, 1991).

Mindell, Earl, and Virginia Hopkins, *Prescription Alternatives* (New Canaan, CT: Keats Publishing, 1998).

O'Mara, Peggy, and Jane McConnell, *Natural Family Living* (New York, NY: Pocket Books, 2000).

Sears, William, and Martha Sears, *The Breastfeeding Book* (Boston, MA: Little, Brown, and Company, 1993).

CHAPTER ELEVEN: USING HERBS TO RESTORE
AND MAINTAIN POSTPARTUM HEALTH

Boone, W.C., and L.W. Wattenberg, "Current Strategies of Cancer Chemoprevention: 13th Sapporo Cancer Seminar," *Cancer Research* 54 (1994): 3315–3318.

Bucci, L.R., "Selected Herbals and Human Exercise Performance," *American Journal of Clinical Nutrition* 272 (August 2000) (Supplement 2): 6245–6365.

Buhner, Stephen Harrod, *Herbal Antibiotics* (Pownal, VT: Storey Books, 1999).

Chan, MMY, et al., "Effects of Three Dietary Phytochemicals from Tea, Rosemary and Turmeric on Inflammation-Induced Nitrite Production," *Cancer Letters* 96 (1995): 23–29.

Davydov, M., and A.D. Krikorian, "*Eleutherococcus Senticosus* (Rupr. and Maxim.) Maxim. (*Araliaceae*) as an Adaptogen: A Closer Look," *Journal of Ethnopharmacology* 72(2) (October 2000): 345–393.

Eschbach, L.F., et al., "The Effect of Siberian Ginseng (*Eleutherococcus senticosus*) on Substrate Utilization and Performance," *International Journal of Sports Nutrition, Exercise, and Metabolism* 10(4) (December 2000): 444–451.

Liu, G.T., "Pharmacological Actions and Clinical Use of Fructus Schizandrae," *Clinical Medicine Journal* (England) 102(10) (October 1989): 740–749.

Melchart, D., et al., "Immunomodulation with Echinacea: A Systematic Review of Controlled Clinical Trials," *Phytomedicine* 1 (1994): 245–254.

Nagabhushan, M., "Curcumin as an Inhibitor of Cancer," *Journal of the American College of Nutrition* 11 (1992): 192.

Pearce, P.T., et al., "*Panax ginseng* and *Eleutherococcus senticosus* Extracts—in vitro Studies on Binding to Steroid Receptors," *Endocrinologia Japonica* 29(5) (October 1982): 567–573.

Rountree, Bob, "Protect Yourself from Colds and Flus," *Let's Live,* December 1998, pp. 61–64.

Rountree, Bob, and Carol Colman, *Immunotics* (New York, NY: G. P. Putnam's Sons, 2000).

Singletary, K.W., "Rosemary Extract and Carnosol Stimulate Rat Liver Glutathione-S-Transferase and Quinone Reductase Activities," *Cancer Letters* 100 (1996): 139–144.

Walker, M., *Olive Leaf Extract* (New York, NY: Kensington Publishing Group, 1997).

Waller, D.P., et al., "Lack of Androgenicity of Siberian Ginseng," *Journal of the American Medical Association* 267(17) (6 May 1992): 2327.

Weed, Susun S., *Wise Woman Herbal for the Childbearing Year* (New York, NY: Ashtree Publishing, 1985).

Zand, Janet, Bob Rountree, and Rachel Walton, *Smart Medicine for a Healthier Child* (Garden City Park, NY: Avery Publishing Group, 1994).

Zhang, L., and X. Niu, "Effects of Schizandrol A on Monoamine Neurotransmitters in the Central Nervous System," *Zhongguo Yi Xue Ke Xue Yan Xu e Bao* [*Acta Academiae Medicinae Sinicae*] 13(1) (February 1991): 23–26.

Resources

PARENTING BOOKS

Darcy, Rahima Baldwin. *You Are Your Child's First Teacher.* Berkeley, CA: Celestial Arts, 1995.

Kabat-Zinn, Myla, and John Kabat-Zinn. *Everyday Blessings: The Inner Work of Mindful Parenting.* New York: Hyperion Books, 1994.

Kitzinger, Shiela. *The Year After Childbirth.* New York: Fireside Books, 1994.

La Leche League International. *The Womanly Art of Breastfeeding.* New York: Knopf, 1998.

Sears, William, and Martha Sears. *The Baby Book.* Boston, MA: Little, Brown & Co., 1993.

Sears, William, and Martha Sears. *The Birth Book.* Boston, MA: Little, Brown & Co., 1994.

Sears, William, and Martha Sears. *The Breastfeeding Book.* Boston, MA: Little, Brown & Co., 2000.

Sears, William, and Martha Sears. *The Fussy Baby Book.* Boston, MA: Little, Brown & Co., 1996.

Solter, Aletha J. *The Aware Baby.* Goleta, CA: Shining Star Press, 2001.

NATURAL MEDICINE FOR
BREASTFEEDING MOTHERS AND CHILDREN

Lininger, Skye, Jonathan Wright, Steve Austin, Donald Brown, and Gaby Gaby. *The Natural Pharmacy.* Rocklin, CA: Prima Health, 1998.

Tierra, Michael. *The Way of Herbs.* New York: Pocket Books, 1998.

Weed, Susun S. *Wise Woman Herbal for the Childbearing Year.* New York: Ashtree Publishing, 1985.

Zand, Janet, Bob Rountree, and Rachel Walton. *Smart Medicine for a Healthier Child.* New York: Avery Publishing Group, 1994.

FUNCTIONAL MEDICINE/CLINICAL NUTRITION

International and American Association of Clinical Nutritionists (IAACN)
16675 Addison Road, Suite 100
Addison, TX 75001
972-250-2829
Fax: 972-250-0233
www.iaccn.org90ccn@msn.com

A professional organization of practitioners of clinical nutrition that provides certification, referrals, educational opportunities and materials, and other services.

Institute for Functional Medicine (IFM)
P.O. Box 1697
Gig Harbor, WA 98335
253-858-4724
www.functionalmedicine.org
An educational organization that provides professional products, publications, and programs to health-care practitioners and patients.

International College of Applied Kinesiology (ICAK)
6405 Metcalf Avenue, Suite 503
Shawnee Mission, KS 66202-4080
913-384-5336
www.icak.org
A professional organization that provides information about applied kinesiology, referrals to AK practitioners, and other services.

American College for Advancement in Medicine (ACAM)
23121 Verdugo Drive, Suite 204
Laguna Hills, CA 92653
800-532-3688
www.acam.org
Provides educational opportunities for health-care professionals and supports research in the field of holistic/preventive/nutritional medicine; maintains a directory of physicians who provide such services.

Dean Raffelock, D.C., Dipl.Ac., CCN
1881 Ninth Street, Suite 210
Boulder, CO 80302
303-541-9019
www.pregnancyrecovery.com

MAIL-ORDER LAB TESTS

Diagnostechs
6620 South 100 92nd Place, Building J
Kent, WA 98032
www.diagnostechs.com
Saliva hormone testing.

Great Smokies Diagnostic Laboratories
63 Zillicoa Street
Ashville, NC 28801-1074
800-522-4762
www.gsdl.com

Performs a wide range of gastrointestinal, immunological, nutritional, endocrinological, and metabolic laboratory assessments. Tests must be ordered by a health-care professional.

Meridian Valley Laboratory
515 West Harrison Street, Suite 9
Kent, WA 98032
253-859-8700
www.meridianvalleylab.com
Twenty-four-hour comprehensive urine hormone testing.

MetaMetrix
4855 Peachtree Industrial Boulevard
Norcross, GA 30092
800-221-4640
www.metametrix.com
Amino-acid panels, fatty-acid panels, and other diagnostic tests.

Pharmasan Labs
375 280th Street
Osceola, WI 54020
715-294-2144
www.pharmasan.com
Laboratory testing services in a variety of areas, including allergy/food sensitivity, clinical chemistry, endocrinology, gastroenterology, and neuroendocrinology.

POSTPARTUM RECOVERY PRODUCTS

Metabolic Maintenance
P.O. Box 3600
Sisters, OR 97759
800-772-7873
www.metabolicmaintenance.com
Nutritional supplements, including custom amino-acid blends based on individual amino- and fatty-acid profiles. Products available through licensed health-care professionals and pharmacists only.

Sound Formulas
1881 9th Street, Suite 210
Boulder, CO 80302
303-541-9019
www.pregnancyrecovery.com
Nutritional supplements to prevent/address common deficiencies that contribute to postpartum problems and delay pregnancy recovery.

Sample Test Results

Laboratory tests to measure an individual's levels of important biochemicals, nutrients, and hormones, and to determine the efficiency of metabolic pathways, can be very helpful because they make it possible to identify precise nutritional deficiencies that can be targeted with dietary changes and with supplementation of key nutrients and hormones. In the pages that follow, you can see what the results of some of the lab tests we have discussed in this book look like.

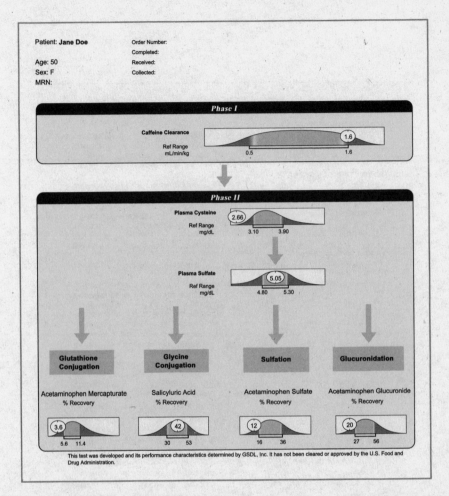

SAMPLE DETOXIFICATION PROFILE

The form above shows a sample result from a comprehensive detoxification profile, which tests for both the availability of nutrients needed for bodywide detoxification and the liver's ability to eliminate toxins when challenged. This patient's results show problems with the detoxification pathway called sulfation. Poor sulfation affects the body's ability to safely dispose of hormones once they have served their purpose. It also has an effect on other body functions, such as cartilage repair and energy production. This test also shows low glutathione conjugation that can impair immune function and low glucuronidation, which can impair detoxification of certain hormones and drugs.

Ordering Physician
Dean Raffelock, DC

Patient: *Jane Doe*
Age: *46*   Sex: *F*

T0040 Fatty Acids - Plasma

Methodology: *Capillary Gas Chromatography/Mass Spectrometry*

#	Fatty Acid	Result		Reference Limits
	Polyunsaturated Omega-3			
1.	Alpha Linolenic (18:3n3)	9	L	15-50
2.	Eicosapentaenoic (20:5n3)	15	L	20-80
3.	Docosapentaenoic (22:5n3)	24		15-35
4.	Docosahexaenoic (22:6n3)	62	L	70-150
	Polyunsaturated Omega-6			
5.	Linoleic (18:2n6)	1063	L	1200-2500
6.	Gamma Linolenic (18:2n6)	9	L	10-26
7.	Eicosadienoic (20:2n6)	6.9		6-16
8.	Dihomogamma Linolenic (20:3n6)	32	L	45-115
9.	Arachidonic (20:4n6)	825	H	300-700
10.	Docosadienoic (22:2n6)	4		≤7
11.	Docosatetraenoic (22:4n6)	7.8	L	8-17
	Polyunsaturated Omega-9			
12.	Mead (20:3n9)	6.8	H	≤6
	Monounsaturated			
13.	Vaccenic (18:1n7)	54		40-120
14.	Myristoleic (14:1n5)	3.2		≤7
15.	Palmitoleic (16:1n7)	93	H	≤80
16.	Oleic (18:1n9)	1600		600-2000
17.	11-Eicosenoic (20:1n9)	6		5-12
18.	Erucic (22:1n9)	3.4		≤7
19.	Nervonic (24:1n9)	45		20-60
	Saturated			
20.	Capric (10:0)	1.9		≤10
21.	Lauric (12:0)	3		≤15
22.	Myristic (14:0)	20		≤100
23.	Palmitic (16:0)	3210	H	1000-2750
24.	Stearic (18:0)	960	H	300-900
25.	Arachidic (20:0)	10		7-17
26.	Behenic (22:0)	30		10-35
27.	Lignoceric (24:0)	52	H	≤30
28.	Hexacosanoic (26:0)	2.3		≤6
	Polyunsaturated Omega-9			
29.	Pentadecanoic (15:0)	8.3		≤15
30.	Heptadecanoic (17:0)	12		≤20
31.	Nonadecanoic (19:0)	2.9		≤7
32.	Heneicosanoic (21:0)	2.8		≤7
33.	Tricosanoic (23:0)	7.8		≤17
	Trans			
34.	Palmitelaidic (16:1n7t)	3.6		≤5
35.	Total C:18 Trans	80	H	≤70
	Saturated			
36.	LA/DGLA	33		12-35
37.	EPA/DGLA	0.47		0.2-1
38.	AA/EPA	17		5-35
39.	Triene/Tetraene	0.026	H	≤0.012

SAMPLE ESSENTIAL FATTY ACID ANALYSIS

The form above shows a sample result from an essential fatty acid analysis, which tests for the amounts and ratios of many key fats found in the blood and tissues. These particular tests reveal a fairly common pattern: The most beneficial fats (DHA, EPA, and GLA) are deficient, while the inflammatory fats (AA and LA) are on the high side. Based on these results, it is possible to prescribe precisely the kinds of good fats this woman's body needs.

Ordering Physician
Dean Raffelock, DC

Patient: Jane Doe
Age: 40   Sex: F

0022 Element Analysis - Erythrocyte
Methodology: Inductively Coupled Plasma - Mass Spectroscopy

	Results	Reference Limits
Essential Elements		
Calcium	9	<= 18.0
Chromium	0.4	0.25-0.80
Copper	0.75	0.52-2.00
Magnesium	32 L	40-80
Manganese	0.12 L	0.25-0.80
Molybdenum	<0.001 L	0.008-0.030
Potassium	1500	1,000-3,000
Selenium	0.07 L	0.12-0.40
Vanadium	0.14	0.10-0.28
Zinc	3.4 L	6.0-11.0
Toxic Elements		
Aluminum	4.2 H	<= 3.0
Cadmium	0.01	<= 0.04
Lead	0.09	<= 0.10
Mercury	0.011 H	<= 0.005

Low Limit / High Limit chart (ppm packed cells): 18.0, 0.25/0.80, 0.52/2.00, 40/80, 0.25/0.80, 0.008/0.030, 1000/3000, 0.12/0.40, 0.10/0.28, 6.0/11.0; Toxic: 3.0, 0.04, 0.10, 0.005

High erythrocyte total calcium has been associated with hypertension, but is not an indicator of your nutritional status of calcium.

Common Adult Supplementation Ranges*	
Chromium	200 - 600 mcg/day
Copper	3 - 5 mg/day
Magnesium	200 - 600 mg/day
Molybdenum	1 - 5 mg/day
Potassium	Fresh Fruits and Vegetables
Selenium	200 - 1000 mcg/day
Vanadium	200 - 1000 mcg/day
Zinc	15 - 60 mg/day

The levels of essential minerals in red blood cells can indicate:
1. Your need for making dietary changes to enhance intake from food sources.
2. Your ability to digest and assimilate minerals.
3. Your need for minerals as food supplements.

Whole grains, beans, peas, nuts, seeds, and shellfish are some of the richest sources of the trace elements. For magnesium, green leafy vegetables and dairy products are also good sources.

*Consult your doctor for specific recommendations and interpretations.

SAMPLE BLOOD MINERAL TEST RESULT
The chart above represents the results of one patient's blood mineral test. The test reveals very high levels of mercury and a pattern of deficiencies in important minerals.

0058 Element - Urine DMSA Challenge

Methodology: *Inductively Coupled Plasma/Mass Spectroscopy*

	Results		Reference Limits	Low Limit	High Limit	
Highly Toxic Heavy Metals						
Arsenic	750		<= 1,000		1000	mcg/day
Cadmium	2.2	H	<= 2.0		2.0	
Lead	11.3	H	<= 10.00		10.00	
Mercury	7.2	H	<= 5.0		5.0	
Potentially Toxic Elements						
Aluminum	25		<= 50		50	mcg/day
Boron	4.70		1.00-20.0	1.00	20.00	mg/day
Essential Elements						
Calcium	62		50-200	50	200	mg/day
Cobalt	64		<= 80.0		80.0	mcg/day
Copper	23.0		10.0-70.0	10.0	70.0	
Chromium	130	H	30-120	30	120	
Iron	733		300-2,000	300	2000	
Magnesium	89	L	100-400	100	400	mg/day
Manganese	14		5-60	5	60	mcg/day
Molybdenum	123		30-200	30	200	
Selenium	742		350-1,000	350	1000	
Vanadium	248		50-350	50	350	
Zinc	962	H	300-800	300	800	

SAMPLE URINE MINERAL TEST RESULT

The chart above represents the results of one patient's urine mineral test. The test pictured here was taken after an injection with a chelating agent, sodium dimercaptopropanesulfonate (DMPS), that pulls these metals out of the body. This sample reveals that the person tested had a toxic load of heavy metals in her body and was flushing a significant amount of heavy metals into her urine.

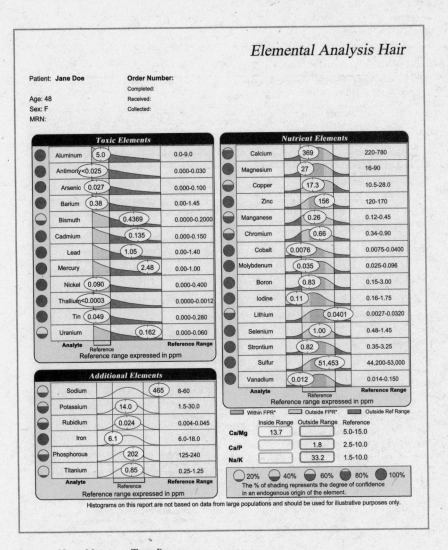

Elemental Analysis Hair

Patient: Jane Doe

Order Number:
Completed:

Age: 48   Received:
Sex: F   Collected:
MRN:

Toxic Elements

Analyte	Reference	Reference Range
Aluminum	5.0	0.0-9.0
Antimony	<0.025	0.000-0.030
Arsenic	0.027	0.000-0.100
Barium	0.38	0.00-1.45
Bismuth	0.4369	0.0000-0.2000
Cadmium	0.135	0.000-0.150
Lead	1.05	0.00-1.40
Mercury	2.48	0.00-1.00
Nickel	0.090	0.000-0.400
Thallium	<0.0003	0.0000-0.0012
Tin	0.049	0.000-0.280
Uranium	0.162	0.000-0.060

Reference range expressed in ppm

Nutrient Elements

Analyte	Reference	Reference Range
Calcium	369	220-780
Magnesium	27	16-90
Copper	17.3	10.5-28.0
Zinc	156	120-170
Manganese	0.26	0.12-0.45
Chromium	0.66	0.34-0.90
Cobalt	0.0076	0.0075-0.0400
Molybdenum	0.035	0.025-0.096
Boron	0.83	0.15-3.00
Iodine	0.11	0.16-1.75
Lithium	0.0401	0.0027-0.0320
Selenium	1.00	0.48-1.45
Strontium	0.82	0.35-3.25
Sulfur	51,453	44,200-53,000
Vanadium	0.012	0.014-0.150

Reference range expressed in ppm

Additional Elements

Analyte	Reference	Reference Range
Sodium	465	8-60
Potassium	14.0	1.5-30.0
Rubidium	0.024	0.004-0.045
Iron	6.1	6.0-18.0
Phosphorous	202	125-240
Titanium	0.85	0.25-1.25

Reference range expressed in ppm

	Within FPR*	Outside FPR*	Outside Ref Range

	Inside Range	Outside Range	Reference
Ca/Mg	13.7		5.0-15.0
Ca/P		1.8	2.5-10.0
Na/K		33.2	1.5-10.0

20%   40%   60%   80%   100%

The % of shading represents the degree of confidence in an endogenous origin of the element.

Histograms on this report are not based on data from large populations and should be used for illustrative purposes only.

SAMPLE HAIR MINERAL TEST RESULT

The chart above represents the results of one patient's hair mineral test. This person's results show high hair levels of mercury, lead, and cadmium.

Ordering Physician				Patient:	Jane Doe
Dean Raffelock				Age: 46	Sex: F

0091 Urine Organix Profile

Methodology: GC/Mass Spectroscopy and Colorimetric

		Result mcg/mg crea		Reference Limits	Low Limit	High Limit
Fatty Acid Metabolism						
(Carnitine & Vitamin B2)						
1.	Adipate	1.5		<= 3.0		3.0
2.	Suberate	2.5		<= 4.0		4.0
3.	Ethylmalonate	3.0		<= 4.0		4.0
Carbohydrate Metabolism						
(Vitamins B1, B3, Cr, V)						
4.	Pyruvate	0.9	H	<= 0.7		0.7
5.	Lactate	35.0	H	4.0 - 30.0	4.0	30.0
6.	α-Hydroxybutyrate	45.0		<= 50.0		50.0
7.	ß-Hydroxybutyrate	30		<= 40		40
Energy Production (Citric Acid Cycle)						
(B Vitamin comp., Q10, Amino acids)						
8.	Citrate	1000		500 - 2,300	500	2,300
9.	Cis-Aconitate	121		5 - 250	5	250
10.	Isocitrate	483		50 - 800	50	800
11.	α-Ketoglutarate	5.2		3.0 - 25.0	3.0	25.0
12.	Succinate	68.5	H	5.0 - 35.0	5.0	35.0
13.	Fumarate	3.5	H	0.2 - 1.2	0.2	1.2
14.	Malate	6.5	H	<= 6.0		6.0
15.	Hydroxymethylglutarate	2.00	H	0.20 - 1.00	0.20	1.00
B-Complex Vitamin Markers						
(Vitamins B1, B2, B3, B5, B12, and Lipoate, Biotin)						
16.	α-Ketoisovalerate	1.5		<= 1.5		1.5
17.	α-Ketoisocaproate	1.5		<= 2.0		2.0
18.	α-Keto-ß-Methylvalerate	2.75	H	<= 1.20		1.20
19.	Methylmalonate	4.7	H	<= 3.0		3.0
20.	ß-Hydroxyisovalerate	26.0	H	<= 20.0		20.0
Neurotransmitter Metabolism Markers						
(Tyrosine & Tryptophan Precursors)						
21.	Vanilmandelate	1.1		0.2 - 2.0	0.2	2.0
22.	Homovanillate	2.5		1.0 - 5.0	1.0	5.0
23.	5-Hydroxyindoleacetate	0.5	L	.08 - 5.0	0.8	5.0
Detoxification Indicators						
(Vit. C, Arg, NAC, Met, Tau . . .)						
24.	p-Hydroxyphenyllactate	0.6	H	<= 0.5		0.5
25.	2-Methylhippurate	1.50	H	<= 1.00		1.00
26.	Orotate	150		<= 180		180
27.	Pyroglutamate	65		<= 80		80
28.	Sulfate	150	L	=> 180	180	
Intestinal Dysbiosis - Bacterial						
29.	Benzoate	3.5		<= 5.0		5.0
30.	Hippurate	601	H	<= 800		800
31.	Phenylacetate	0.9		<= 1.2		1.2
32.	Phenylpropionate	0.8		<= 1.2		1.2
33.	p-Cresol	155	H	<= 150		150
34.	p-Hydroxybenzoate	7.5	H	<= 5.0		5.0
35.	p-Hydroxyphenylacetate	85	H	<= 50		50
36.	Tricarballylate	3.1	H	<= 1.8		1.8
Intestinal Dysbiosis - Clostridial						
37.	Dihydroxyphenylpropionate	3.0	H	<= 0.9		0.9
Intestinal Dysbiosis - Yeast/Fungal						
38.	Tartarate	75		<= 80		80
39.	Citramalate	6.5		<= 10.0		10.0
40.	ß-Ketoglutarate	2.00	H	<= 1.00		1.00

Creatinine =84 mg/dl

SAMPLE ORGANIC ACID TEST RESULT

The chart above represents the results of one patient's organic acid test, a urine test that can provide a very good picture of overall nutritional status, metabolic activity, detoxification processes, and intestinal health.

Ordering Physician
Dean Raffelock, DC

Patient: *Jane Doe*
Age: 46   Sex: F

Healthcare Guide Based on Positive Indicators From Organix™

Strength of Insufficiency Indicators ⟶

B-VITAMINS	NONE	SLIGHT	MODERATE	SEVERE
B-complex vitamins			50-100 mg each/day	
Biotin		5 mg 2x/day		
L-Carnitine	0			
Niacin			250 mg/day	
Pantothenic Acid	0			
Riboflavin		50-200 mg/day		
Thiamin			100 mg 3x/day	
Vitamin B12			1000 mcg 3x/day	

Multiple B vitamins may best be taken as a comprehension B complex formula

MINERALS				
Chromium	0			
Iron		18 mg/day		
Magnesium & Calcium		200-500 mg/day		
Manganese				15 mg/day
Vanadyl sulfate	0			

ANTIOXIDANTS				
CoQ10				100-300 mg/day
Lipoic acid		50-150 mg 3x/day		
N-Acetylcysteine	0			
Vitamin C		50-100 mg/kg body wt/day		
Vitamin E		400 IU/day		

AMINO ACIDS (BCAA=Branched chain amino acids)				
α-Ketoglutarate		500-1000 mg/day		
Arginine	0			
BCAA	0			
Glutamine				2000 mg 3x/day
Glycine		300-600 mg 3x/day		
Taurine		500 mg 2x/day		
Tyrosine &/or Phenylalanine	0		1000 mg 2x/day	

PROBIOTICS				
Lactobacillus spp.				3-6 caps/day
& other probiotics				
Saccharomyces boulardii				2-4 caps/day

COMMENTS
- Antifungal agents recommended.
- Avoid simple sugars and disaccharides.
- Eat a high fiber diet (prebiotic support).
- Tyrosine is contraindicated for patients taking MAO inhibitors.

No parts of this laboratory report are intended to take the place of a qualified health care professional's advice. This information is intended to help educate and aid interpretation or review potential healthcare options.

No attempt has been made to specify dosages. All amounts shown are based on adult repletion levels.

SAMPLE RECOMMENDATIONS BASED ON ORGANIC ACID TESTING

The table above represents recommendations for a nutritional supplement program to correct deficiencies identified through organic acid testing (see page 282).

Comprehensive Digestive Stool Analysis

Patient: **Jane Doe**

Order Number:
Completed:

Age: 27
Received:
Sex: F
Collected:
MRN:

Digestion

		Reference Range
Triglycerides	2.1	<= 3.1 mg/g
Chymotrypsin	44.9	1.4-36.8 U/g
Valerate, iso-Butyrate	4.9	0.8-20.1 umol/g

	Inside	Outside	Ref. Range
Meat Fibers	None		None
Vegetable Fibers	Rare		None - Few

Absorption

		Reference Range
Long Chain Fatty Acids	4.4	<= 15.0 mg/g
Cholesterol	0.8	<= 3.2 mg/g
Total Fecal Fat	8.0	<= 16.6 mg/g
Total SCFAs	70.9	23.8-165.4 umol/g

Microbiology

Bacteriology

Beneficial Bacteria
Lactobacillus species I NG
Escherichia coli N
Bifidobacterium I NG

Additional Bacteria
alpha haemolytic Streptococcus N
gamma haemolytic Streptococcus N
Citrobacter freundii P
Klebsiella pneumoniae P

Mycology

Candida albicans P

Metabolic Markers

		Reference Range
n-Butyrate	6.8	2.4-39.4 umol/g
Beta-Glucuronidase	4,336	937-4,500 U/g
pH	6.1	6.0-7.2

SCFA distribution

		Reference Range
Acetate	44	46-72 %
Propionate	24	12-34 %
n-Butyrate	12	10-32 %

Immunology

	Inside	Outside	Reference Range
Fecal Lactoferrin	Negative		Negative

Macroscopic

Color	Brown		Brown
Mucus	Negative		Negative
Occult blood	Negative		Negative

*NG = No Growth   N = Normal flora   I = Imbalanced flora   P = Possible pathogen

Dysbiosis Risk Index

12

Optimal   Slight   Moderate   Severe

Intestinal Permeability

Lactulose Percent Recovery	1.3
Ref Range %	<= 0.8 ... 2.0
Mannitol Percent Recovery	48
Ref Range %	5 ... 30
Lactulose/Mannitol Ratio	0.03
Ref Range	<= 0.07 ... 0.20

This test has been developed and its performance characteristics determined by GSDL, Inc. It has not been cleared or approved by the U.S. Food and Drug Administration.

Commentary

Results are dependent on renal function. The mannitol determination has been corrected for concentration variability in the pre- and post-challenge urine collections by determining the creatinine concentrations and relating these to the mannitol determinations. In circumstances of significant renal insufficiency with low urinary creatinine concentrations in both the pre- and post-urine specimens, corrections for mannitol concentration variability using creatinine determinations cannot be done.

Lactulose and mannitol recoveries are elevated, suggesting an overall increase in permeability both between and through the intestinal epithelial cells. The elevated lactulose reflects increased paracellular permeability (between the cells), which can result in macromolecules, toxins, and antigens crossing the intestinal barrier into the lymph and circulatory systems, a condition termed "leaky gut." These particles increase the load on the body's detoxification system and may stimulate immune reactivity. Increased lactulose recovery has been associated with food allergy, inflammatory bowel disease, arthritis, and other inflammatory conditions.

The elevated mannitol reflects increased transcellular permeability (through the cells) which may result in the passage of small antigens across the mucosal barrier, thereby triggering an immune response.

SAMPLE CDSA TEST RESULT

The figure above represents the result of one patient's comprehensive dietary stool analysis (CDSA) with intestinal permeability testing. It revealed that she had a high level of *Candida albicans* and inadequate beneficial bowel flora—and, indeed, this woman was suffering from the typical symptoms this imbalance can cause, including chronic fatigue, depression, sugar cravings, and weight gain. Test results like these are often seen after a round of antibiotic drugs, which kill off the probiotic bacteria that keep yeast growth in check.

Permissions and Credits

Figure 3.2 on page 50 is adapted from a figure in *Clinical Nutrition: A Functional Approach* by Jeffrey Bland, Ph.D. (Gig Harbor, WA: Institute for Functional Medicine, 1999). Used by permission of the Institute for Functional Medicine.

Figure 3.4 on page 56 is adapted from a figure from *Brain-Building Nutrition: The Healing Power of Fats and Oils* by Michael A. Schmidt, Ph.D. (Berkeley, CA: North Atlantic Books, 2001). Used by permission.

Figure 4.1 on page 67 is adapted from a figure in *Clinical Nutrition: A Functional Approach* by Jeffrey Bland, Ph.D. (Gig Harbor, WA: Institute for Functional Medicine, 1999). Used by permission of the Institute for Functional Medicine.

The guidelines for modified elimination diet on page 171 are adapted from material in *Clinical Nutrition: A Functional Approach* by Jeffrey Bland, Ph.D. (Gig Harbor, WA: Institute for Functional Medicine, 1999). Used by permission of the Institute for Functional Medicine.

The Many Roles of Progesterone on page 200 is adapted from *What Your Doctor May Not Tell You About Premenopause* by John R. Lee, M.D. Used by permission.

The figures on pages 277, 281, and 284 were supplied by the Great Smokies Diagnostic Laboratory. © 2001 Great Smokies Diagnostic Library. Used by permission.

The figures on pages 278, 279, 280, 282, and 283 were supplied by MetaMetrix, Inc. Reproduced with permission of MetaMetrix, Inc.

Index